Yoga for Health and Vitality

No matter what age you are, you can achieve a healthy and active life by following the exercises in this book. Clearly and carefully explained, with simple line illustrations and diagrams, by one of Europe's leading yoga experts, the exercises cater not only for the young and athletic, but also for those who are unfit or overweight or who suffer from the major and minor ailments that accompany modern urban life, such as dietary and muscular disorders, heart trouble, dyspepsia, constipation, tension, anxiety and depression, headaches, breathing trouble or poor circulation.

Using methods described in these pages, the author has helped hundreds of pupils and patients to lead a richer and fuller life. An 11-year-old girl who had stopped growing at the age of 5 gained twelve inches in a year. A woman of 26 who had faded to a pathetic skeleton of 81 lb thanks to partial paralysis of the colon recovered her former health and vitality. One patient critically ill after a spine operation regained the use of his limbs. Another with an acute thyroid condition found that haemorrhages ceased after a course of breathing and relaxation exercises. And, perhaps most remarkable of all, a woman who weighed 270 lb and who had been bedridden for many years regained a normal figure and an active way of life after losing nearly 90 lb in 11 months.

Included in the book are special exercises for the middle-aged and elderly, for those who are under- or over-weight and also for pregnant women. There are no reliable statistics to show how many cases of high blood pressure, haemorrhoids or stomach ulcers have been cured or relieved by yoga, but Max Kirschner has treated so many cases successfully that there can be no doubt about the effectiveness of his methods – and he has been especially successful in treating patients suffering from a tilted pelvis, a complaint which can cause severe discomfort or even cripple, which is known to afflict many millions of people and which often goes undiagnosed.

The author is one of the few experienced teachers who have made a special study of remedial yoga and of the ways in which yoga can foster vitality and prolong an active and healthy life. This book will be used with benefit not only by those who suffer from specific complaints, but also by all those who are willing to devote even as little as twenty minutes a day in order to achieve greater health and happiness.

MAX KIRSCHNER was born and educated in Munich. After fifteen years as a tobacco planter in Sumatra, for ten years he ran a dairy farm near Simla, then worked for the Indian government introducing modern methods to protect crops all over northern India. Thanks to yoga he recovered from a severe illness and since then has devoted his life to teaching, experimenting and lecturing.

LILIAN K. DONAT is well known as a writer and journalist. Since visiting India in 1968 she has spent most of her time teaching and writing about yoga and runs the London School of Yoga.

Yoga for Health
and Vitality

M. J. KIRSCHNER

Translated from the German by Lilian K. Donat

LONDON   GEORGE ALLEN & UNWIN LTD
Ruskin House   Museum Street

This translation © George Allen & Unwin (Publishers) Ltd 1977

ISBN 0 04 149042 8 hardback
     0 04 149043 6 paperback

Originally published in German as
Die Kunst sich selbst zu verjüngen
© 1958 Agis-Verlag, Baden-Baden

Printed in Great Britain
in 10 point Plantin type
by Butler & Tanner Ltd
Frome and London

Contents

Preface

Dr Gunter Schultz and his wife, Dr Sophie Schultz, have helped with advice and information to create this book. Occasionally they also enabled me to use my own methods and experience for their patients. I therefore dedicate this book to them with gratitude.

To show what can be achieved with Yoga breathing and exercises, the following cases seem to be suitable illustrations.

Case 1. The little dwarf

One day Dr Sophie Schultz called me to see a new child at a school which was under her medical care. She knew the medical history of this pretty 11-year-old girl who had stopped growing at the age of five when she was three foot three inches tall. Since then nothing had succeeded in stimulating her growth. I showed her various postures which act on the pituitary gland, such as the headstand and deep relaxation. We had only two sessions altogether and the child grew, according to measurements taken at school, about twelve inches during the next two years. As the family moved away, I lost sight of her.

Case 2. Eczema

Another time Dr Gunter Schultz asked me to visit one of his patients. She had been seen by many specialists over the last six years and was pronounced the worst case of eczema in Munich. Although married and only 26 years of age, she lived alone in a dreary room leading the life of a recluse for fear of showing herself to other people. She had lost hope of ever leading a normal life again. Dr S. had warned me not to show my shock when seeing her. Despite this warning I must confess that I was not prepared for the sight which struck me when she opened the door.

She looked like a walking skeleton; her weight was a mere 81 lb. Her head was entirely bald and she had neither eyebrows nor eyelashes. Her mouth was covered in scabs. Her room had a foul atmosphere which indicated a serious malfunctioning of her bowels. She told me that she only defecated once a week and judging by her walk it was obvious that one leg was shorter than the other. She informed me that her dermatologists considered this as a congenital fault.

There and then I made her do one of the best exercises for a tilted pelvis, namely the Spiral, and in a short while this divergence righted itself and both her legs were equally long.

I supposed that hers was a case of a partial paralysis of the rectum which caused a continuous self-poisoning. My hunch proved to be correct. She was able to defecate the next day and started eating again.

Altogether I gave her seven lessons in two weeks. The scabs began to fall off. I then asked Dr S. to remove her from that terrible room, hoping that a change of surroundings would accelerate her recovery. Her family then sent her to Ischia where she went for walks and went bathing in the evening, still avoiding people as much as possible. When she returned after two months the eczema was gone although she still had scars on her face. Her eyebrows and lashes had grown again and her head was covered by a red fuzz of hair. I shall always remember the way she looked at me when I saw her again. After that I never saw her, but I was told that she had divorced her husband and left Munich.

Case 3. Bernd, a peasant boy

The 9-year-old boy had been brought to a children's hospital with severe constipation, and in a serious condition. From Christmas to the month of April various experiments had been tried but all that could be done for him were enemas. My insistence that it was possible to educate the peristalsis was received with great scepticism by the doctors, but as nothing else had succeeded so far, I was allowed to re-educate Bernd. The first thing that struck me was that his breathing was wrong as he contracted the abdomen during inhalation. I managed to make him change this bad habit during our first session. Three days later, after our second session, he had already succeeded in moving his bowels twice, and by the end of the week he managed to defecate three times a day. Many members of the hospital staff stood around watching the boy performing his exercises.

After this, the doctors decided to have a special Yoga class for themselves in the hospital.

Case 4. Mr 'X'
One day a deeply upset stranger arrived on my doorstep and implored me to come immediately with her to see her husband who was lying critically ill in a private clinic. As he was in great pain he had agreed to have a spinal operation but she was afraid that he might then be doomed to a life in a wheelchair. In her despair, she begged me to talk him out of the operation. This, I felt, would be medically unethical but in view of her distress I agreed to at least accompany her to the clinic.

When I saw the patient I found that one leg was not only one whole inch shorter than the other but was also severely atrophied and was totally without sensation from the knee downwards. I decided to try something; if it did not succeed, there was still time for the operation. His wife stood guard at the door while he practised 'the spiral'. I then advised him to refuse the operation for the time being, to continue to practise the spiral and to try to walk as much as possible. He did this and two days later happened to meet his surgeon on the stairs. The surgeon was naturally intrigued by this sudden change for the better and not in the least annoyed that the operation had been cancelled. However, he did express the desire to meet the man who had effected the improvement.

When I went to meet him in his private surgery, I noticed that he had trouble to rise from his chair. When I suggested that I might be able to help him he agreed to lie down on the carpet, and in this case too the spiral did its work and corrected his twisted pelvis. He was well pleased and we parted as friends.

Mr 'X', by the way, was cured completely within a year and was able to go on several long journeys, including one to India where he joined a school of meditation.

Case 5. The Bleeding Lady
One day a beautiful young woman of about 35 years came to me with the following complaint: for the last three and a half years she had been suffering from haemorrhages which usually lasted from ten to twelve days during which period she was con-

fined to bed. After an interval of five or six days the bleeding started again. She had consulted many doctors, had had several D. and C.s, injections and pills. She was at the end of her tether.

I had the impression that her thyroid was overworked and suggested exercises to increase the action of the pituitary. (See 'Taming the Thyroid'.) There are certain practices in Yoga which can stimulate the endocrine glands. We began with headstands, breathing exercises and long periods of relaxation. As I had hoped and expected, it helped. After the first two sessions which took place in one week, she stopped haemorrhaging. It would appear that her body now was able to produce its own oestrogen and now, four years later, no further haemorrhages have occurred.

Case 6. Resi – the peasant girl from the mountains
Four years ago her father confessor brought her to me and she had trouble to climb up to the first floor. She was then 49 years old and weighed approximately 270 lb. For the last fifteen years she had been a patient in a Kneipp clinic, living on her small pension. Most of the time she had to stay in bed. Her kidneys hardly worked and she had thick varicose veins and suffered from permanent backache. On her calf was a visible mark of thrombosis.

My first suggestion was that she had to lose weight; as she was a strong-willed person, she managed to lose approximately 77 lb in ten months. When she had achieved this she wanted, for the first time in sixteen years, to buy herself a dress off the peg. She found a suitable garment at a greatly reduced price – but it was still a little too small for her. Bravely she decided to drop yet another 10 lb. She managed this in four weeks and proudly bought the pretty dirndl.

Her vast improvement came to the notice of the authorities and a board of doctors decided that she no longer qualified as an invalid pensioner. This meant that her pension was discontinued but Resi never worried – she had exchanged it for her long-lost health. She now works as a chambermaid at the same clinic in which she had been a patient for so long. On Sundays and during her holidays she goes up into the mountains. She told me that during one of her holidays she went to visit a doctor who had known her during her bad days. He looked at her in silence, then he shook his head and said: 'It is unbelievable what can be achieved with Yoga.'

TAMING THE THYROID

As has been shown in some of the previous cases, it is possible to influence two of the endocrine glands which produce hormones, namely the pituitary and the thyroid. One reads in medical textbooks that the glands of the endocrine system should function like a well-trained orchestra. In speed and pitch they must correspond with each other. If the conductor (the pituitary gland) slows down, the big drum (represented by the thyroid gland) takes over and creates havoc in the whole orchestra. The result is nervous overstimulation which seems altogether much more frequent in the West than in the East. An overactive thyroid is easy to recognise: the throat becomes enlarged and the eyes protrude. A Greek doctor with whom I discussed this during a visit to the Acropolis Museum showed me a head of a prominent victim of this overstimulation: Alexander the Great, with the unmistakable features of a hot-tempered man of action with protruding eyes and swollen throat, a portrait of one of the most aggressive personalities of world history. 'Without his type of thyroid he would never have been able to conquer half of Asia,' remarked the doctor.

When the thyroid overfunctions it releases a certain hormone into the circulation which, even in small quantities, constricts the blood vessels, increases the pulse rate and tenses the muscles. If the pituitary is unable to deliver the special hormone which counteracts the other, the state of stress becomes permanent, with the result we see so often – the restless, aggressive man, unpopular at work and at home. Forever on the move, he cannot find rest even in his sleep.

Yet this hormonal disturbance can be corrected by such exercises as the headstand, alternate breathing and relaxation. Other remedies are the transmission of the life force called Prana in India. Cases I and V show that the body is able to produce the necessary hormones in a short time and without the assistance of drugs. My medical friends agree with me that a real cure can be achieved with the help of Yoga.

THE EIGHT LIMBS OF YOGA

HATHA-YOGA (Affirmation of Life)		RAJA-YOGA (Withdrawal from Life)
		(8) Superconsciousness (*Samadhi*)
		(7) Meditation (*Dhyana*)
Window →		
(3) Relaxation (*Pratyahara*)		(6) Concentration (*Dharana*)
(2) Breathing Practices (*Pranayama*)		(5) Disciplines (*Niyama*) Purity Contentment Austerity Self-Study Devotion
(1) Postures (*Asana*)		(4) Restraints (*Yama*) Non-Hurting Truthfulness Non-Stealing Chastity Non-Coveting
Aim: Rejuvenation		Aim: Extinction of self

I

Introduction

In my working profession as an agricultural adviser and during my stay of thirty years in India, I met many of the representatives of all classes and particularly of the Kshatriya (warrior) aristocracy, with whom I often spent the cool hours of the night in peaceful conversation on roofs and terraces. I was told of traditions of the courts and of famous clans and families, and I was shown many postures. This sometimes happened on the battlements of a castle, in camps in a clearing of the Terai, a rich plain at the foot of the Himalayas. Once I talked to the manager of a factory in a house between railway lines and smoking chimneys. There were also contacts in trains and resthouses, at universities and research institutes where I met many interesting people. A *sadhu* (good one or mendicant) introduced me to headstands on a mountain meadow amidst broken statues of a ruined Hindu temple. All my teachers have received me kindly and answered my questions openly.

What is often mentioned in this book as the 'Indian opinion' is the sum total of the cross-section of advice and explanation and the reservations and warnings which I heard. Those warnings which appear in this book constitute for me an important part of the pragmatic against the dogmatic philosophy of Yoga. Most of my friends stressed the necessity of remaining inside one's own limitations and recognising what one can and what one cannot do. This was Yoga without the personal cult of the *guru* (lit. the 'heavy one', spiritual guide), and without the claim of holiness which the dogmatic school considers its prerogative.

I am most grateful to my teachers, to my colleagues in the West and to the many books which deal with the subject of Yoga. I have learnt from all of them, including my pupils.

WESTERN YOGA BOOKS

Many Western presentations of Yoga make a sharp distinction between Raja-Yoga (Raja – 'royal') and Hatha-Yoga (Hatha – 'force'). Hatha-Yoga is the path of Yoga in which, amongst other things, physical postures and breath control are taught. They consider Raja-Yoga to be mainly a mental discipline and Hatha-Yoga a system of physical processes leading up to higher mental exercises. This is not quite correct and ignores the common ground of both. Far from being a substitute for those who cannot take up the mental disciplines, Hatha-Yoga is a perfectly valid path to the high goal of all types of Yoga aiming at the awakening of man's full potential. Another shortcoming of many Western Yoga books is their lack of modesty and the discrepancy between their often ambitious intentions and the actual readiness of the readers to put the theories into practice. There is also too much armchair Yoga in the West. A good book should inspire the reader to take up the practice of Yoga without overstimulating his hope or fantasy, nor should it discourage him by making excessive demands on his time or energy.

THE ESSENCE OF TRUE YOGA

Every student should be taught to recognise the difference between right and wrong Yoga while still a beginner. I got an answer to this question as the result of a very unpleasant experience with a group of pilgrims who attacked and plundered a train at a small station between Calcutta and Patna. (In India, thousands of pilgrims are part of the scene on all stations where they wait patiently in the hope of boarding some train.)

Although I myself suffered no personal loss, I was horrified to see the pilgrims attack and smash the train and plunder whatever they could carry away. I wondered why these obviously religious people could become so violent for no reason visible to me. Weeks later I had to go to the same station in order to cross the Ganges. On the other bank of the river was a small temple where I sat down next to the priest who had just finished his meditation. I then remembered the incident and told him about the peculiar 'pilgrims' I had met. He supposed that they only had wanted to travel for a few stops to be able to bathe in the Ganges; in his opinion they became violent because something had upset them.

'Who else but a pilgrim would travel on the holy night of the full moon?' he said with silent reproach. I was slightly embarrassed and asked who, in his opinion, was a genuine pilgrim. 'I am sure God would prefer a simple pilgrim who crosses the river in order to meditate in my temple rather than one who would cross mountains and valleys and travel for 2,000 miles to reach the holy lake of Manassarowa but, on the way, would enter gambling and drinking houses. The genuineness of a pilgrim cannot be measured by the length and difficulty of his journey, Sahib, but by the sincerity of his intentions.'

Here I had my reply to the question of true or false Yoga. Acrobatics and difficult postures do not make a true Yogi. One who, within his limitations, modestly strives each day towards a certain goal—he alone follows genuine Yoga.

THE AIM

Sincerity and modesty demand the choice of an aim which is within your grasp. The first step is to achieve a triple cleaning of the accumulated poisons in the body by practising breathing, postures and relaxation. This means that our Hatha-Yoga is first and foremost health education which will become an experience and a sensation manifesting itself in the form of rejuvenation. This does not exclude a certain heightening of our consciousness or awareness, which is what many people expect from Yoga. Our path, too, leads to this goal but it is reached at the end and not at the beginning of the journey. An educational system resembles a skyscraper: one enters at the ground floor and climbs up by one's own effort—not by shooting up in a lift.

Once we accept the disciplines of breathing, postures and relaxation we should stop misusing our body and mind. Usually we rush from one task to the next without pause; we drive ourselves by our ultra-competitive attitude and when our strength fails we resort to drugs. All for the sake of keeping up with time.

In comparison with this way of life one can say that the Indian recharges his spiritual batteries in the intervals between his activities. He is capable of contemplative concentration which is difficult for the Westerner who thinks that one can achieve everything by using the will for action.

WHAT CAN THE 20-MINUTE YOGI EXPECT?

It is good to know that the authenticity of Yoga is relative and determined by the limitations of the student and his philosophy. When we contrast dogmatic and pragmatic Yoga we can see at a glance that what would be a sin for a Brahmin, is permitted to a Kshatriya. The pragmatic method does not expect any religious vows such as following the five rules of *yama* for example. (Yama – 'discipline' comprising unconditional non-injury (*ahimsa*), truthfulness, non-stealing, greedlessness and chastity.)

The dogmatic Yogi who has sworn celibacy will practise special postures to sublimate his sexual energies. Those who want to escape from the wheel of rebirth are not interested in rejuvenation.

The dogmatic school aims at a lofty and distant goal – *samadhi* (a state of heightened consciousness in which the mind becomes identified with the object of contemplation). The student pays a high price to reach it by practising celibacy, poverty and by living for years a life of renunciation and service. This is not for everybody, and the average person leading an average life in the Western sense cannot expect to reach this goal. The first prerequisite for any kind of ritual such as prayer and meditation is inner purity. Meditation is not denied to my readers, but this book will take them only as far as the threshold. For this reason it is not necessary for the student to learn the Lotus posture (*padma-asana*). This posture can be painful and takes a long time to learn for the Westerner who is accustomed to sitting on chairs. Many people have been put off Yoga by the pedantic attitude of a dogmatic book which places this feat at the beginning of all instruction. My book aims at opening the door to Yoga – not closing it.

YOGA FOR ACTIVE PEOPLE

One cannot expect too many sacrifices or changes from a beginner, and one certainly cannot make too many demands on his limited time. In the West things are very different from India where every monk or hermit finds people who will feed him all his life, thus allowing him unlimited leisure. According to an age-old Indian tradition this promises good fortune to the benefactors.

This book only requests two periods of 20 minutes each per day, two blankets and a cushion, and a real desire to learn the right approach to Yoga. The first 20 minutes are used for performing the *asanas* ('postures') before breakfast, while the second 20 minutes are needed for relaxation either during the day or evening.

TO HELP THE STUDENT

Once a student has become interested in pragmatic Yoga he must be taught to help himself, beginning with the removal of his inhibitions. There is no reason why Yoga should only be a monastic school of renunciation and world negation. It can become a friendly and positive way of life which does not demand unreasonable self-sacrifices. The little plasures of life can still be enjoyed: this particularly applies to the corpulent and elderly among my readers for whom life is already sufficiently difficult. They can so easily be discouraged if they are expected to practise a kind of Yoga which lies outside their province; a pedantic teacher or a perfectionist could quickly lose some of his stiff or corpulent pupils by expecting too much from them.

THE INDIRECT MASTERY OF THE VEGETATIVE FUNCTIONS

Man has by and large three enemies: time, gravity – and himself. Time is a cosmic fact; its advance makes us grow older without our being able to change it. Gravity is also responsible for the ageing of man, but in Yoga this same gravity is utilised for the process of rejuvenation.

Premature ageing has five causes: one is wear and tear and the other four are neglect, displacement of organs, self-poisoning and worry. The following diagrams show that not only mechanical but also emotional influences affect the digestion by causing spasms of the intestines. This is a daily occurrence known to every doctor.

Vitality can be acquired through a method which the student can practise by himself; he then will be able to correct displacements of the inner organs and remove spasms through the practice of the Contemplative Breath. 'Emotions such as fear, anger or jealousy can cause temporary contractions. Intestines affected in this way look like chains of large beads on an X-ray. Single sections are distended by fermentation and gases. These sections or pockets can collect poisonous waste.'[1] A smoothly working peristalsis (forward movement of the intestines) is an important part of the education for vitality which can be learnt.

Normal position of intestines. Easy functioning and passage; one of the secrets of vitality. Undisturbed peristalsis.

PASSAGE

constriction here

Enlarged abdomen owing to increase of weight alters the position of the intestines. Flatulence and constrictions are the results. Peristalsis is badly affected.

[1] From a book by the author. By courtesy H. Wimmer, Munich Grunwald.

THE CONCEPT OF VITALITY

Vitality is a composite concept. Roughly speaking it consists of three components: genetic inheritance, environmental influence and the individual urge for self-fulfilment. Man acquires his inheritance at the moment of conception; this inheritance can have positive as well as negative traits. The environmental influence begins already in the womb and dominates a child for many years. The drive for personal fulfilment begins with growing up, and the adolescent strives for confirmation of his personality and for recognition through his knowledge and his achievements. All this can act like the fuel in a rocket.

Vitality varies with each individual and normally reaches its climax around the twenty-fifth year of life and sometimes begins to diminish a few years later. Theoretically one could draw two curves, one for the physical and the other for the mental ups and downs. It should be possible to measure the peak of the first curve by testing the capacity of the individual under physical strain. For the mental curve one might perhaps try to assess how far the personality can cope with responsibility without losing the creative impulse and without showing signs of breakdown. For most people the physical and mental climax is not far removed from the beginning of ageing. This is taken into account in the modern industrialised nations, when it is thought that men around 40 have already lost a good deal of their creativeness. It also means that the course of the curve determines the fate of man – and not the other way round.

EDUCATION FOR VITALITY

It is a great tragedy that millions of people pass two-thirds of their lives on the descending curve. Once a stone has been thrown, both its course and the place where it lands are predetermined. The trajectory of the stone depends entirely on the following criteria: impetus, shape and weight of the stone, and aerodynamics. At this point begins the lesson of how to increase vitality. Here lies the vast area of unused possibilities where Yoga should come in. Dogmatic Yoga has not advanced beyond scholastic studies and is not concerned with the problems of our times. It calls into question the possibility of evolution. On the other hand, as this book is trying to show, there are many ways in which the course of evolution can be assisted.

THE PSYCHO-SOCIAL REVOLUTION

This is the name Sir Julian Huxley has given to the great transformation which in the twentieth century has influenced the realms of intellectual life, religion, education, politics and economy. Evolution is an effort to direct fate by adaptation or improvement. It is possible for us, with the help of Yoga, to determine our vitality curve and make it rise to unexpected heights.

An essential prerequisite of the psycho-social revolution is, according to Huxley, that man is free to examine and discard traditional knowledge and to formulate his own concepts in a favourable mental environment. As pragmatists (as opposed to dogmatists) we must have the freedom to explore and replace old and inadequate concepts with new and better or more suitable ones. To one of these concepts belongs the professional woman and mother, hardly known in Indian life, who has achieved her rightful place in society. In many Yoga schools, seminars and courses, women form the majority of the participants. Pragmatic Yoga enables women to make life easier for handicapped and elderly family members, by introducing them to 'Yoga over Sixty'. In some continental countries there are over ten million old people of which less than half are men. Yet these men need two to three times as much medical care as women in the same age-group. It would be a great achievement if these circumspect women could keep their male counterparts out of wheelchairs.

TASKS OF PRAGMATIC EXPLORATION

There are innumerable ways in which pragmatic Yoga can investigate and help. The possibility of correcting the overfunction of the thyroid through activating the pituitary gland is one of those. *Prolapsus recti* can, in many cases, be remedied with Yoga without the need of an operation. The cleansing of the sinuses relieves, and sometimes cures, respiratory diseases. It seems strange that the appropriate exercises do not belong to the curriculum of our schools. Perhaps this is the case because many Yoga books talk of cure instead of correction, which annoys the medical profession.

There are still many other unexplored questions. During my eighteen years of practice I have learnt that the experience of warmth during relaxation cannot only be explained by improved circulation due to the dilation of the capillaries which is caused by a hormone in the pituitary gland. In addition to this there is yet a 'second warmth' which has a completely different effect; it is felt like a flowing or a penetrating radiation, moving in waves; this can be intensified at certain points and then acts like a foreign body. With experience this heat can be directed to various parts of the body to relieve tension or even pain.

II

Breathing

Rejuvenation starts with the correction of breathing. Breathing, properly understood, is not just the inhalation and exhalation of air; other factors are involved. It is also of the greatest importance to breathe with the whole instead of with only a part of the lungs and much depends on how the air is directed into and out of the lungs. Furthermore, the posture in which one breathes and the kind of thoughts that accompany the breath are important. Only when all this has been taken into account, breathing turns into a real experience.

First of all the hygienic side of breathing: if we compare the lungs with a sponge, saturation happens during inhalation and the squeezing out of the sponge corresponds to exhalation. This is a good picture because the lungs are in fact a sponge-like organ. Imagine air as a perishable liquid – such as milk – which can go stale when it is retained and not expelled. The air we breathe is, of course, not stale but it contains enough impurities which, if they remain in the lungs, can behave in the same way as fermenting milk.

The lungs hang in the thoracic cavity; though they can be squeezed, they can never be completely emptied. Exhalation is, at best, only an incomplete squeezing out of the sponge. With each breath there is a residue of about one litre of air left in the lungs. (This, by the way, is a vital necessity, as otherwise the lungs would collapse.)

To come back to our comparison with milk; the residual air could be called the equivalent of yesterday's milk remaining at the bottom of the bottle. Although this comparison is not ideal, it has the advantage of helping one to visualise a sponge in whose holes and openings the perishable contents can lead to the formation of phlegm. If nothing is done about it, this residue could become a seat of infection.

It is not surprising to find diseases of the lungs caused by residual air and it also explains why immobile, bedridden patients have to be turned over several times a day; if they were lying on the back for several days, the fermentation could cause pneumonia. In other words, if the residue is allowed to settle down, it leads to fermentation which leads to inflammation. When the patients are moved or massaged, a certain exchange of fresh and stale air takes place, preventing inflammation.

The human thorax has an elastic floor, the diaphragm. This floor is so constructed that it lowers with the inhalation, letting the lungs expand; with the exhalation it curves up into the thorax, with the result of squeezing out some of the residue. This action of the diaphragm is called abdominal breathing. No air will actually enter into the abdomen but the abdomen blows up and deflates like a balloon.

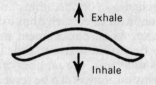

OUT WITH THE RESIDUE

Inner cleanliness demands that there should be as little stale air as possible and that one gets rid of the residue several times daily through 'squeezing the sponge'. The best postures for this are the Shoulderstand (*viparita-karani*) or the Headstand (*shir-sha-asana*). With these inverted postures one can achieve a degree of cleanliness of the lungs which is not possible when standing, sitting or lying. It does not mean that every corpulent person must immediately do the Headstand; on the contrary, he should practise other exercises which will take a little longer to get results – but which are equally efficient in giving him relief.

WHAT ABOUT THE HEART?

The heart will be raised and lowered during the more or less ' energetic breathing movements. As corpulent people often have weak hearts, they should have a medical examination before attempting such practices. Generally speaking, the right exercises are beneficial, since the heart can take this kind of massage. It has even been shown that breathing exercises can improve, if not cure, various heart diseases. In any case it is better to seek a doctor's advice before starting with the practice.

BREATH AS CLEANSER AND ENERGISER

Speaking in physical terms, breath is the extractor of an important raw material which it introduces into the metabolism; from a mixture of gases a certain percentage of oxygen is extracted without which man cannot do. If one compares the process of breathing with that of digestion, the latter resembles a one-way street. The breathing process, on the other hand, is more like a dual carriageway with a fast-moving transport of gas shuttling in and out. The mechanics of our breathing are such that breath changes its direction in an uneven rhythm using the same gate for entrance and exit. As all nourishment must pass through the stomach so our breath has to traverse the lungs. Now if you compare the lungs to a bank, the number of serving counters determines how many customers can be served simultaneously. Breath transports a quantity of unsorted gases into the bank (the lungs) and pumps out the material which is handed over at the counters. It is rather like a transport firm which is not particularly interested in the contents of the boxes it carries.

The alveoli (minute bubbles which compose the bulk of the lung tissue) have chemically active linings which extract the valuable oxygen and reject the rest. Inside the alveoli this is hastily handed over to a red corpuscle which has been waiting eagerly for this nourishment and which gives in exchange a small quantity of the waste product carbon dioxide. A rough picture of this complex process is that the carbon dioxide has to be eliminated at the same speed as it is produced, since otherwise it turns into poison (lactic acid) when it accumulates in

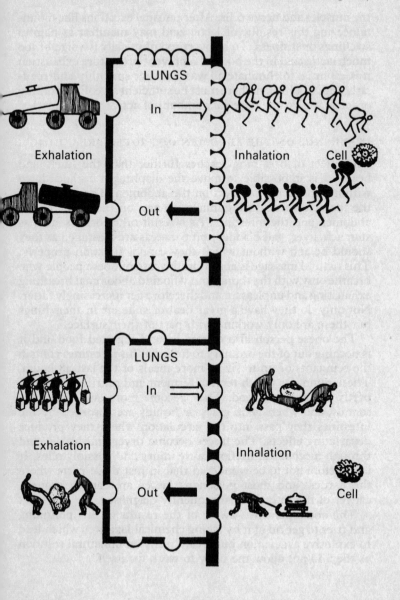

LUGNS

In

Exhalation

Out

Inhalation

Cell

LUNGS

In

Exhalation

Out

Inhalation

Cell

the muscles and nerve cells. After unusual exertions like moun-
taineering this residue of lactic acid may manifest as painful
swellings or stiffness. To be overtired physically is a sign of too
much lactic acid in the body. To prevent premature exhaustion
it is essential to eliminate all waste matter smoothly and regularly and, in addition, there must be sufficient alveoli in working
order as well as the necessary amount of active red corpuscles.

INFLUENCE ON THE ABDOMEN OF PROPER BREATHING

The effect of breathing reaches further than the lungs and
heart: it is impossible to move the diaphragm up and down
without producing an effect on the abdomen. The increase of
the thoracic space during inhalation acts on the inside of the
abdomen and the intestines. As a result other organs such as
stomach, liver, gall bladder and pancreas are massaged as they
should be and without which they cannot function properly.
This natural massage is absent in the case of obese people who
breathe only with the thorax and who find abdominal breathing
exhausting and unpleasant and therefore get increasingly fatter.
Not only do they have a great deal of stale air in their lungs
but these are only working with part of their surface.

The obese person also carries around digested food and it
is nothing out of the ordinary to find that his intestines contain
the remnants of up to six or more meals of the last 48 hours.
These remnants which tend to ferment and putrify, consist of
partly decomposed food. They become more and more poisonous, and when toxic gases or liquids are absorbed by the
intestines they pass into the circulation where they produce
devastating effects. The faeces become dryer and harder and
through mechanical friction cause injury and possibly piles. It
is therefore not to be wondered that in just those parts where
the hardest and most poisonous faeces are carried around,
cancer of the intestines is frequently diagnosed.

The obese person is aware of the results of this poisoning
and tries to get rid of it by taking chemical laxatives which lead
to explosive evacuation but create really an unnatural solution
as they do not allow the body to work for itself.

IN THE BEGINNING IS THE BREATH

Breathing exercises which move the diaphragm upwards and downwards produce a dual cleansing effect: above, they squeeze the lungs and free them from their residue; below, they cause the peristalsis to cleanse the intestines and so start the gradual cleansing of the body. It is not only in the intestines in which an obese person carries the collected waste matter – he carries it also in kilos of fat and fluid in the various organs, muscles and tissues.

Good respiration brings back mobility of the lungs and the abdomen. It is mainly the abdomen which makes the obese person feel that he is carrying around a heavy load which acts like a dead weight. Here it is worth mentioning that nobody is expected to use abdominal breathing *all* the time. It should be practised only for a few minutes several times a day, preferably in a lying position. Without proper breathing it is impossible to lose weight and keep it down.

YOGA BREATH IS MORE THAN AN INTAKE OF AIR

Yoga differs from other systems of physical exercises in that it stresses the mental awareness and conscious direction while performing the exercises. This is noticeable even at the beginning. The first step to help oneself begins with an exercise which we shall call the *Contemplative Breath*.

Lie on a blanket on the floor with a pillow under the head and with knees bent and touching each other while the feet are apart. This position is particuarly suitable for an overweight person as he usually has a hollow back which makes lying down

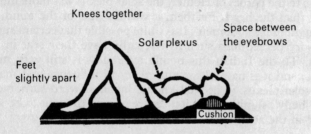

Knees together

Solar plexus

Space between the eyebrows

Feet slightly apart

Cushion

on the floor painful. Now start abdominal breathing – as you inhale only through the nose let the abdomen rise as far as possible. Exhale slowly, again through the nose, and allow the abdomen to sink in. Repeat this for two minutes. Most people will sense a feeling of warmth in the solar plexus when practising this technique calmly and with concentration. (Solar plexus means 'sun plait'. It refers to the major nerve centre situated in the region of the stomach.)

THE SOLAR PLEXUS AND THE AUTONOMIC NERVOUS SYSTEM

The feeling of warmth mentioned above can only be described approximately. The beginner has a slight sensation of flowing warmth which spreads perhaps over parts of the abdomen and gives him a feeling of alleviation and release. With practice this warmth will become more evident. In other words, daily practice of the Contemplative Breath will enable the beginner to become familiar with his solar plexus. In most people's minds the solar plexus is associated with boxing, as a hit in this area often results in a knockout. Emotional reactions are also felt in this part. Fear, disappointment or annoyance seem to produce a contraction, often expressed in such phrases as 'I cannot stomach it', or 'I feel sick when I see him'.

The unpleasant and painful reactions of the solar plexus due to emotional upsets are well known. Duodenal and other ulcers of frustrated people are almost proverbial and so is the internal cramp or colitis of nervous women. It may help in regaining one's awareness of the body when one realises that the solar plexus played an important role in the life of primitive man. Even to the heroes of Homer, the solar plexus was more important than the head; for them it was the seat of the mind, 'he thought in his abdomen'. It is quite possible that certain supersensory perceptions such as telepathy have their seat in this area. To the Indian this bodily awareness is still very much alive, and it is natural for him to try to influence and master the solar plexus. (The well-known Japanese word *hara*, meaning 'belly', signifies the vital centre of man thought to be situated in the abdomen.)

The solar plexus is part of the autonomic nervous system which does not normally respond to orders. It can be compared to a telephone exchange with special lines which can only be used by the authorities. The autonomic nervous system is in charge of all the important things which function during sleep such as breathing, digestion, the work of the glands, metabolism and the healing of wounds. This 'telephone line' can only be used by those who have learnt how to use it. The Yogi, for instance, has learnt not to order but to 'ask' the autonomic nervous system to help him. One of the means of approach to this nerve centre is the Contemplative Breath during which one makes use of the different temperatures of inhalation and exhalation. The Contemplative Breath is a kind of warm and cool breath also acting on areas which are inside the head behind the eyes. We shall call these spots the 'trigger points'. Others are situated at the back and above the throat, in the upper sinuses and in the area of the hypophysis. This gland lies deep inside the head yet it is only divided from the upper sinuses by a thin partition of bone. Besides this, there are nearby the upper two ganglias of the sympathetic nerve.

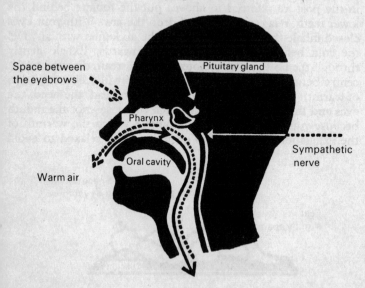

Space between the eyebrows

Pituitary gland

Pharynx

Oral cavity

Sympathetic nerve

Warm air

The action of the 'cool inhalation' aims at the sympathetic nerve while the 'warm exhalation' probably starts in the sinus area which has an opening pointing towards the back. Dr Walter Scheidt, Professor of Anthropology at the University of Hamburg, writes: 'At the back of the upper wall of the pharynx just where with normal nasal inhalation the air hits the wall of the pharynx, there lie, a few millimetres below the mucous membrane, the two upper nerve ganglia (*cervicalia superiora*). This area becomes cooled with inhalation and warmed with exhalation. . . .

. . . every inhalation thus represents a stimulation of the upper nerve ganglia.'

What interests us here is the 'collectedness' or focus on a particular point which, in yogic literature, is referred to as the 'space between the eyebrows', also known as 'triple peaks' (*trikuta*). This focusing happens in a relaxed mental attitude, not during tense concentration. While in this state one should relax the face as well, slightly dropping the lower jaw.

The important thing is to try to experience this for yourself. Make sure that your clothes are not restricting and lie down in the posture referred to above; put the tongue behind the lower teeth, relax your face and drop the jaw. With your eyes closed inhale through the nose, fill the abdomen with air, feel the cold behind the eyes and look inwards. Exhale gently through the nose in a conscious flowing stream directed to the centre between the eyebrows; there you will feel a sensation of warmth which spreads through the forehead, the head, the eyes and the cheeks. Exhale through the nose – not the mouth because you would bypass the point to which the warmth of the exhalation is directed. The jaw is only relaxed to avoid

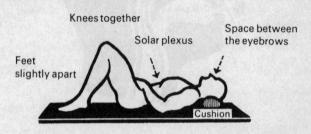

Knees together

Solar plexus

Space between the eyebrows

Feet slightly apart

Cushion

clenching the teeth. Relax – sink. Inhale – cold, exhale – warm. In and slowly out – again in and slowly out. The slower and the more flowing your breath, the greater and the more distinct the sensation of warmth. This warmth moves like a wave with every exhalation, and we will refer to it as the 'warm impact' which can soon be felt in your solar plexus.

WHY BREATHE THROUGH THE NOSE

Before we continue to speak about directing the warmth it must be mentioned that breathing through the nose is essential for man's general wellbeing. This applies particularly to those living in a cold climate where the temperatures sinks to freezing point. It is a shock to the body when you fill the lungs with icy-cold air inhaled through the mouth, since it contracts the throat and the air passages. Inhalation through the nose both filters and warms the air considerably before it reaches the lungs. When the cool air drawn in through the nostrils touches the 'trigger points' inside the head, a sensation of wellbeing which will spread to the other parts of the body will be felt in the solar plexus. The student will soon recognise how he can prolong this cool flow by breathing slower. Then a whole series of new experiences will begin.

DIRECTION OF WARMTH AS A MEANS OF RELIEVING CONTRACTION

The art of conscious 'abreaction' is a contribution to rejuvenation which is one of the aims of many Hatha-Yoga students. (This German word used in Psychology has become a technical term in English. It means the release of pressure built up as a result of unpleasant experiences.) The art of 'abreaction' consists of both a breathing technique and a mental process. One could call it the essence of Yoga: not only are physical exercises performed in slow motion but it is essential to participate mentally as well. Understanding is a part of thinking – and the more one understands, the easier the process. If we understand how a cramp starts we shall understand how to relieve it. Cramp is an involuntary contraction which cannot be consciously relieved but which can be 'approached' through concentration on the 'trigger points' which react to the cool and warm flow of the breath. These points are also able to send directions to other centres, for example to the solar plexus, where a sensation of warmth is created to relieve the cramp. It can be directed to most parts of the body and it is comparatively easy to channel it to reach the traverse intestine and to the descending branch of the colon. If during this practice one puts the right hand on the abdomen covering the liver and gall bladder, the warmth will be felt there, whereas if it is placed on the left side of the abdomen, covering the descending branch of the colon, one will feel a gurgling and flowing which indicates the release of a cramp.

WARMTH AS ENHANCED CIRCULATION

Consider the wellbeing of a sleeping child, lying in its cot with rosy cheeks and a warm body. Our own bodies which have never quite forgotten this sensation are always longing for the well being resulting from a good circulation. Contrast this state with the euphoria caused by drugs; this is a kind of artificially induced wellbeing which does not correspond to the true condition of a person. The natural contentment of the sleeping child is caused by the dilation of the capillaries – a state which can be recreated in an adult using the Contemplative Breath. The fine network of the capillaries can open or close and therefore increase or decrease the nourishing amount of oxygen. This mechanism belongs to the involuntary nervous system which does not respond to any orders from the individual.

When the capillaries in the intestines or anywhere else in the body are constricted, an unpleasant state of tension is produced or vice versa. The same state can also be caused by emotions such as fear or anger. To counteract this effect we have to practise calm concentration combined with breathing which will invite the sympathetic nervous sytem to relax the state of tension, indicating that we have the means to normalise circulation by dilating the blood vessels. This technique aims at the indirect mastery of the autonomic nervous system. For example, the bear is a master of this technique: He has the gift of producing a negative direction of warmth which lasts for months. By lowering his body temperature to 6°C, he sinks into a cataleptic state in which breathing and other physical functions cease almost entirely; this is known as hibernation. In the spring he starts with the positive direction of warmth, when he raises his temperature and wakes up to normal life.

Indian Raja-Yogis can perform similar feats. It has happened that a Yogi has been buried alive for up to forty days and was taken out not much worse for wear. Little is known about the breathing techniques used by them. Presumably the retention of the breath after exhalation plays an important role which helps to reduce all bodily functions to a minimum, as in an animal during hibernation.

This voluntary 'hibernation' demonstrates an amazing mastery of the autonomic nervous system. In comparison with this, it seems a small feat when we try to direct some warmth into our cold feet, an arthritic hip or a painful knee. Before we go any further we shall try to experiment with the laying-on of hands.

EXERCISE

Return to the relaxation posture and breathe slowly through the nose as before. Cover the region of the solar plexus with your hands on either side and if it makes you feel more comfortable, put cushions under the elbows. If the room is cold, cover yourself. Now start breathing consciously, noticing the difference between warm and cool. Inhale – abdomen out, exhale – abdomen in, relax your face, think of the space between the eyebrows and behind your eyes. First feel the warmth there. Slowly it also becomes warm under your hands. Listen: Can you hear the gurgling in your abdomen? If so, then this will be your first conscious direction of warmth. You have learnt something which will always be of use to you. If you feel nothing, please be patient and continue to practise.

PREVENTION OF COLDS

Although Yoga cannot protect you from flu, a Yogi under normal circumstances does not catch cold. He prevents it by doing breathing exercises aimed at the cleansing of nose, throat and sinuses.

Indian ideas of cleanliness go much further than the Western concept of hygiene. The cleansing of the skin, pores, mouth and teeth is not sufficient, since according to the Indians the germs of infection can be hidden inside the nose, throat and sinuses. They therefore also insist on a complete elimination of digested food not later than twelve hours after a meal. A conscientious Indian following this method would not dare to enter a temple without having had an evacuation in the morning. In the strict sense he is 'unclean' and hence unacceptable. For the same reason he would not attend a wedding since he would be afraid of bringing bad luck to the young couple.

The Indians are also more 'dust conscious' than we are. Living in a very dry continent where, during the hot season, dust rises up to 2,000 metres, penetrating even the houses up in the Himalayas, he practises sniffing up water with salt or bicarbonate of soda. Holding the water in the hollow of his hand he draws it up with the nose and spits it out. This method is not always to be recommended in colder climates. On the other hand *bhastrika* ('bellows'), a breathing exercise, is an absolute necessity. This can be performed either sitting or kneeling. Before going further with breathing exercises, a few words about posture.

THE LOTUS POSTURE AS A DETERRENT

It is a popular misconception of Western readers that the Lotus posture (*padma-asana*) is an essential in the practice of Hatha-Yoga. In actual fact this posture is used mainly for meditation in Raja-Yoga. The Indian, with or without Yoga, spends his whole life sitting on the floor, and therefore this posture comes naturally to him. The Westerner who spends most of his life sitting on chairs naturally does not find the Lotus posture so congenial. Of course the student is free to learn it if he so wishes, but the one posture which he really needs is the easier Thunderbolt posture (*vajra-asana*).

BHASTRIKA IN THE THUNDERBOLT POSTURE[1]

Fold your blanket as thickly as possible, kneel and sit down on your calves; your big toes are together and your heels apart with the top of the foot flat on the blanket. If this is too difficult forget it for the moment and practise while sitting on a chair. This kind of *bhastrika* consists of exhaling through one nostril, closing it, and inhaling through the other nostril. Put the right index finger at the bridge of the nose, close the right nostril from below with the thumb, lean slightly forward and exhale through the left nostril. Now close the left nostril with the thumb, inhale right, exhale left, inhale right, exhale left. With the inhalation you straighten up and with the exhalation you bend forward. Then change the direction of the breath, beginning to exhale left and inhale right. Practise this for 30 seconds during your daily 20-minute Yoga. (This technique is more often called alternate breathing or *surya-bheda* 'piercing the sun'.)

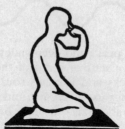

WHAT IS THE AIM OF THIS EXERCISE?

It is inner cleansing of the axillary cavities and the sinuses; both of these will be blown out with the impetus of the exhalation as if one were using a fine spray from a scent bottle. One can increase the effect in the case of purulent inflammation by bending the head sideways; if the left side is infected one closes

[1] This is Kirschner's own way of *bhastrika*, which is normally considered to be a forceful exhalation.

the right nostril and bends the head to the right for the exhalation. This helps also in the case of sinus trouble.

BREATH AND EMOTIONS

Consciously experienced breath is more than physical cleansing because it also influences our emotions. Everybody knows how he reacts to fear or anger. The heart beats faster and a cold sweat breaks out. Graphically expressed, this shows as an angry zigzag line. The rising line stands for inhalation and the falling for exhalation. An angry person does not think of his breath and so this diagram shows a picture of unconscious breathing.

Angry person's
breathing

Equally unconscious is the calm and flat breathing of a woman who sits quietly and knits, and hers is a curve of softly flowing

Calm person's
breathing

breath without high peaks and deep valleys. These two curves are identical with the state of mind of the people concerned. To the ancient Greeks and Romans soul and breath were as one, and the words they used – *pneuma* and *spiritus* – meant both soul and breath. The sharp zig-zag of the breath of the emotionally excited person can be evened out into the flowing wave of a tranquil mind with the help of the Contemplative Breath; the tremor of fear can be turned into calm courage; thus the positive result of conscious breathing is the control of the rhythm of the breath.

CONCENTRATION ON THE RHYTHM OF BREATH

When we tune into the wavelength of our own breath we become conscious that it is not we who breathe but 'it'. The rhythm is not something that we command, but an experience invited by expectation and inner collectedness. In our mind we connect a wavelength with an even, unfluctuating movement. Practically speaking, this means that every inhalation and exhalation should be equal to the previous one.

Everybody's personal rhythm depends on his physique and the degree of practice, and it is essential to discover one's individual rhythm or 'wavelength'. With practice and experience this rhythm becomes slower in time and has a calming effect on the psyche. The alleviating of emotional disturbance is almost instantaneous with the practice of the Contemplative Breath and Complete Breathing.

Comparative Diagrams

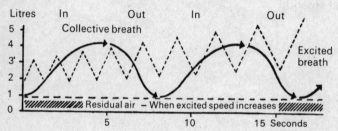

Complete Breath while kneeling (beginners)

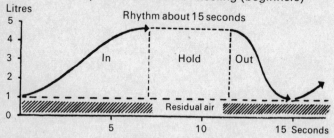

THE COMPLETE BREATH IN THREE STAGES

Western medicine accepts three stages of inhalation: first abdominal, then thoracic and finally clavicular, breathing with the upper lobes of the lungs. The Complete Breathing is performed in a single slow movement comprising all three stages. This is done by rising from the starting position shown in the first diagram. The following diagrams depict the exercise as executed by four types of students: the normal, the athletic, the obese and the aged or weak. The most important thing to remember when doing these breathing exercises is that one must be constantly aware of the coordination of breath and movement. If it happens that by mistake you exhale whilst doing the inhalation movement or vice versa, you should stop the exercise and start again from the beginning. Do not breathe slower or retain the air any longer than is comfortable. Both inhalation and exhalation must be done through the nose and the breath must be distributed in such a way as to ensure that breathing is even and smooth.

Breathing Exercises

FOR AVERAGE PEOPLE

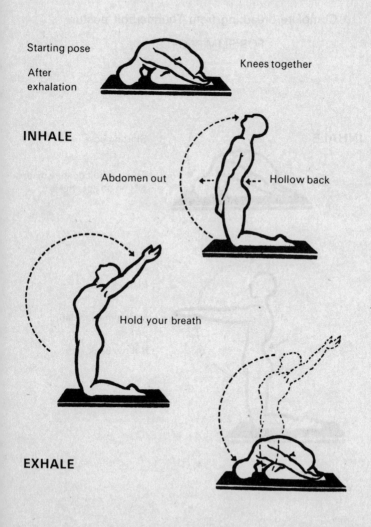

Starting pose

After exhalation

Knees together

INHALE

Abdomen out ← → Hollow back

Hold your breath

EXHALE

COMPLETE BREATHING IN THUNDERBOLT POSTURE

Important: Inhalation and exhalation are performed through the nose and represent an even flow, achieved by the regular distribution of the breath.

Complete breathing from Thunderbolt posture

FOR SLIM PEOPLE

INHALE

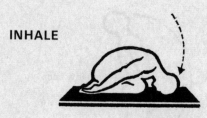

1. Starting pose

   Thunderbolt posture means sitting on your heels

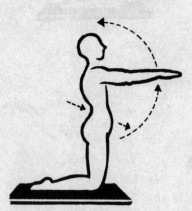

2. Rise up

   Abdominal inhalation

   Hollow back

INHALE

3. Thoracic breath which raises the abdomen slightly

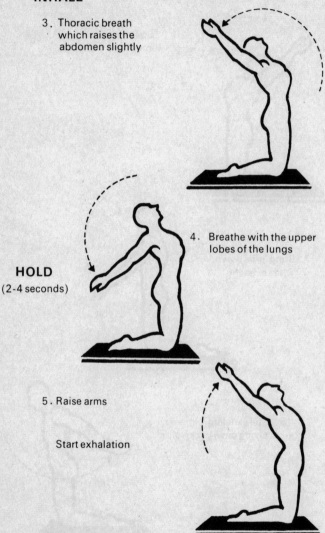

4. Breathe with the upper lobes of the lungs

HOLD

(2-4 seconds)

5. Raise arms

Start exhalation

EXHALE

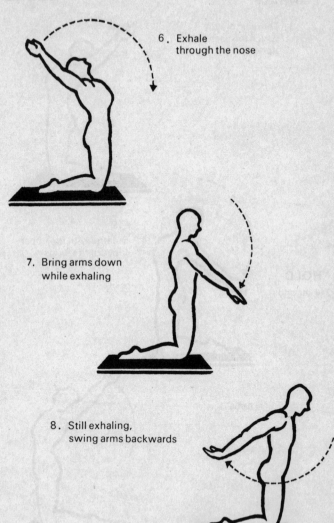

6. Exhale
through the nose

7. Bring arms down
while exhaling

8. Still exhaling,
swing arms backwards

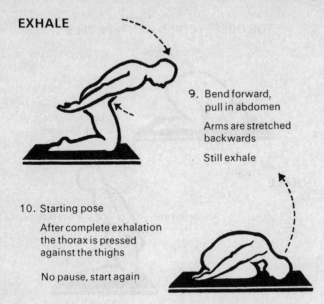

EXHALE

9. Bend forward,
   pull in abdomen

   Arms are stretched
   backwards

   Still exhale

10. Starting pose

    After complete exhalation
    the thorax is pressed
    against the thighs

    No pause, start again

This Complete Breathing should be practised six times first thing in the morning, preferably with the window open. It is essential that the student performs the first abdominal breath correctly; this means that the abdomen must protrude and the hollow in the back must be accentuated. Only by doing this can the diaphragm be raised to ensure the correct execution of the Complete Breathing. Furthermore, the movement of the arms is very important. During the thoracic breath the out-stretched arms form a half circle upwards, with the palms pointing forwards and the arms at each side of the head.

The inhalation with the upper parts of the lungs is completed by turning the arms sideways and backwards with the palms turned upwards. Then pause: Obese, aged or weak *hold no pause*.

FOR OBESE (CORPULENT) PEOPLE

Preparation

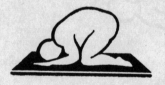

After exhalation,
support yourself
on the forearms

INHALE

Abdomen out   Hollow back

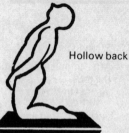

Hold
(2-4 seconds)

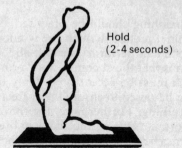

EXHALE

Return to starting pose

S-L-O-W-L-Y

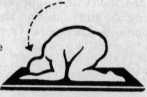

COMPLETE BREATH FOR OBESE PEOPLE

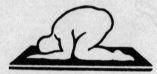

1. After exhalation, bend forward and support yourself on the forearms

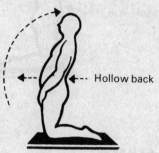

2. INHALE

Abdomen out ← ← Hollow back

3. INHALE

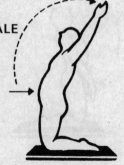

Arms up

Abdomen in

4. INHALE

Swing arms backwards

Hold (2-4 seconds)

Palms upwards

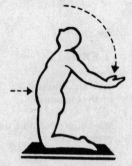

5. EXHALE

Arms up

Abdomen in

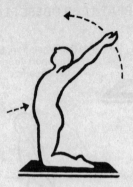

6. EXHALE

Swing arms down

Pull abdomen in

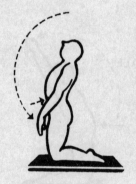

7. EXHALE

Support yourself
on the forearms

Maximum exhalation through
pressing down

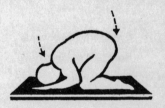

FOR UNCOORDINATED OR CLUMSY PEOPLE

Preparation

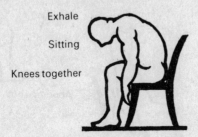

Exhale

Sitting

Knees together

INHALE

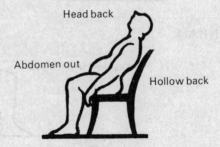

Head back

Abdomen out

Hollow back

EXHALE

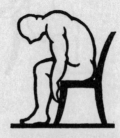

Press thighs
against abdomen

COMPLETE BREATH FOR
UNCOORDINATED OR CLUMSY PEOPLE

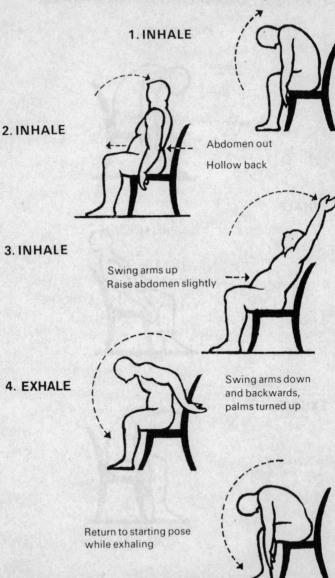

1. INHALE

2. INHALE

Abdomen out

Hollow back

3. INHALE

Swing arms up
Raise abdomen slightly

4. EXHALE

Swing arms down
and backwards,
palms turned up

Return to starting pose
while exhaling

It is advisable that the student does the three phases of inhalation in a single flowing breath and that he is very conscious of the even distribution of the inflow of the air, particularly during the first phase. Always breathe through the nose. The time for all three phases together should take five to eight seconds.

BREATH RETENTION (KUMBHAKA)

After full inhalation, stop at first for one second in the posture shown as No. 3 in diagram. More will be said of this breath retention later.

EXHALATION

The exhalation also follows through the nose. It is a slow outpouring of air in controlled quantities. The body remains stretched, only the arms move while the air is exhaled. The arms describe a circle of 360 degrees, and they are brought backwards with the palms upwards. Then bend forwards and draw the abdomen in while exhaling; bow and place the trunk on the thighs, squeezing out the rest of the air. Be careful not to inhale in between and do not remain in this position but start immediately with the next inhalation.

ONCE MORE CONCENTRATION ON THE FLOW

Although it is difficult to focus your thoughts on a single point, it is relatively easy to follow the rhythmical repetition of a wave. Everyone loves to watch the breaking of the waves on the sea shore, being fascinated by the approaching and receding of the

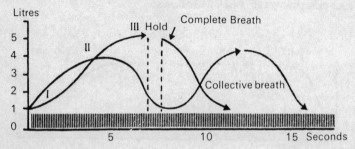

waves. The same applies to the rhythm of the breath. Imagine
the inhalation as if it were an approaching wave while the
exhalation is the wave which flows away from you. For the
beginner this simile will be helpful when he is practising the
Contemplative Breath while lying on his back. Once the rhythm
has been established in this posture he can transfer it to the Complete Breathing sitting in the Thunderbolt posture.

The waves drawn in this diagram have a rhythm of eight
seconds (Contemplative Breath) and thirteen seconds (Complete Breathing) respectively. This, however, is only a suggestion, and one can practise shorter or longer waves according
to one's liking and ability. The rhythm of the Complete Breathing can be prolonged by a second per week according to the
following table:

Initial Rhythm of first and second week　　third week fourth week etc.

			third week	fourth week etc.
Inhalation (*puraka*) phases I, II and III				
	= 8 secs	9 secs	9 secs	9 secs
Pause (*kumbhaka*)	= 1 sec	1 sec	2 secs	2 secs
Exhalation (*recaka*)	= 4 secs	4 secs	4 secs	5 secs
	= 13 secs	14 secs	15 secs	16 secs

As you see, the rhythm increases gradually and slowly until
it reaches to thirty seconds. Be aware that exaggeration can be
dangerous. It is quite sufficient to do about six Complete
Breaths to begin with ($1\frac{1}{2}$ minutes). Beginners are especially
warned not to use the rhythm normally prescribed in Yoga textbooks which is meant for the experienced Yogi. This rhythm,
counted according to the pulse beats, is 1 : 4 : 2. Translated into
seconds this wave looks as follows:

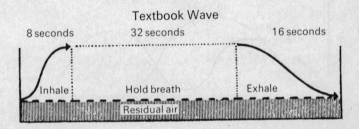

Textbook Wave

8 seconds　　　32 seconds　　　16 seconds

Inhale　　Hold breath　　Exhale

Residual air

In comparison with the thirty-two seconds (retention) plus sixteen seconds (exhalation), the eight seconds of inhalation are extremely short. I therefore suggest that the follower of the 20-minute Yoga does not retain the breath for more than six seconds. On the other hand the whole process can be extended to forty or fifty seconds, provided the student feels no discomfort and prefers the slow rhythm. Once more it should be emphasised that there is no pause in the Contemplative Breath which should flow smoothly from full inhalation into exhalation.

APPLICATIONS IN EVERYDAY LIFE

The Complete Breathing can be practised standing or sitting at any time of the day without taking any particular posture or moving the arms as shown in the previous exercises. It is an invaluable help to the practice of self-control which will come automatically as you continue to use the Complete Breathing. This will enable you to check your automatic reactions to the irritations and disappointments of everyday life. If there is no time for the 20 minutes of relaxation during the day or if you are feeling particularly low, practice the six Complete Breaths as you did in the morning.

In great heat a breathing exercise called *shitali* ('cool') has a cooling effect. This is done by rolling the tongue into a tube lengthways, while sucking in the air through the mouth; the exhalation is done through the nose. When repeating it six to ten times one realises that the lungs are also an organ for the regulation of the body temperature.

It takes some time until the student experiences the flow of *prana*. (According to the Indian sources, *prana* penetrates and sustains the whole body. Its external manifestation is breath. Lack of *prana* in certain parts of the body causes illness. On the other hand, it is possible to charge the body or parts of it with *prana* and thus cure illnesses or prevent them.) *Prana* is not yet measurable with our scientific instruments, and for the time being the only way to convince oneself of its existence is by taking up yogic breathing exercises.

THE MARK OF VITALITY

Most mature adults have an equal lung capacity in terms of size and intake of air, yet their vitality can differ to a marked degree. The difference lies in the fact that some people's lungs have a great number of active alveoli, while others have allowed many of them to degenerate through bad breathing habits. The man of action is more youthful as he is capable of quick regeneration. The prematurely ageing man, on the other hand, has allowed part of his lung area to atrophy, but it is still possible to reactivate these areas by forming new alveoli. (A fact which, at present, is not recognised by doctors.)

The number of alveoli is constantly increasing in the lungs of young people, although they decrease in number when the lungs are not fully used. By practising *pranayama* (*Pranayama* – 'control of the life-force') systematically, the alveoli in hitherto neglected parts of the lungs regenerate, thus increasing the active area of the lungs.

According to Indian opinion, with every breath we absorb not only oxygen but also another life-giving element which is not exhaled. It is called *prana* (lit. 'life'). The name and theory are unimportant. What counts is that as a result of his painstaking efforts, the student can experience a constant intensification in himself. This is a sure sign that he is on the way to rejuvenation (often even needed in young people). It is best begun with rhythmic abdominal breathing.

BREATH HYGIENE AS CANCER PREVENTION

The latest progress in cancer research indicates that a cancer cell is a degeneration of a former normal cell. This degeneration is caused by chronic damage of the cell respiration. The degenerated cell does not have its former oxygen combustion, but the blood sugar turns into lactic acid through fermentation and this transformation can be created artificially by the deprivation of oxygen.

This should not give you the impression that practising breathing exercises is an instant cancer cure. On the other hand, one could argue that an obese person breathing shallowly is more likely to invite cancer. This fact is confirmed by statistics. Obese people are five times more cancer-prone than slim people, and therefore have to pay higher insurance rates. There also are five times as many obese diabetics and eight times as many people with heart disease amongst the obese. They also often have a tendency to get varicose veins.

But there is still help for them. The Contemplative Breath can be practised even by the plumpest person. Everybody can lie on his back and permit his thoughts to ride on the waves of his breath. For this reason this chapter will finish with a more intensive form of the Contemplative Breath.

CONTEMPLATIVE BREATH WITH FOUR BARS

Lie down on your blanket with a cushion under the head (not under the shoulders and the nape of the neck). The knees touch and the heels are slightly apart. The small of the back is lowered to the ground so that it lies flat on the blanket. The hands frame the solar plexus.

Inhale (through the nose) – the abdomen rises, exhale (through the nose) – the abdomen sinks. Imagine a wave and watch how it approaches and then retreats again. Breathe smoothly. There should be no jerking.

Now here is something new: One – inhale slowly into the abdomen. Two – continue inhaling into the chest. Three – exhale with the abdomen. Four – exhale with the chest. Phase Four is the shortest part of the exhalation and One is the longest. We will call this the Four-Bar Breathing. You will notice immediately that this is like the movement of a wave. Bar one and two, the wave approaches you. Bar three and four, the wave recedes. As you breathe in, imagine and feel an inflow of strength which accumulates. With the exhalation feel the flowing away of all that is undesirable: fear, anger and anxiety.

III

Detoxication

CONTROL YOUR BOWELS

Hatha-Yoga begins with inner cleanliness. The Raja-Yogis, too, practise this with the help of special exercises and methods. An Indian Yogi may consume about 100 grams of rice, a little milk, honey and fruit per day; this is his entire nourishment between times of fasts. Before a Raja-Yogi goes into deep meditation he will make sure that his body is completely free from digested food. To cleanse his stomach, he will sometimes swallow about 25 metres of a thin cotton cloth soaked in water; when drawn out the cloth is supposed to have removed impurities from the stomach. He also can, with the help of his sphincter muscles, give himself a colonic irrigation while standing in a river. Only after this thorough cleansing would he consider himself worthy to enter higher realms. It is equally important for a student of Hatha-Yoga to dedicate time and effort to master the functioning of his own digestive system to the point where he is able to eliminate at will.

CONTINUOUS SELF-POISONING

Most of us suffer from a constant overloading of the digestive system. We eat three to four times a day, while an Indian has only two main meals. Our frequent meals demand constant work from both stomach and intestines. According to Indian concepts the digestion of a meal should not take more than seven hours – a maximum of two hours in the stomach and five hours in the small intestines. The latter extract the nutritional elements from the food and leave waste matter, i.e. faeces. These are then moved into the large intestines and slowly towards its exit.

There is no reason that this waste should be carried for more than eight hours after a meal, but there are many reasons for eliminating as quickly as possible, because after twelve hours the faeces become toxic. The degree of toxicity increases quickly and after forty-eight hours in the intestines the faeces become a very dangerous source of poison. The dissolvable toxins are drawn into the circulation; the development of gases takes away the elasticity of the intestines and leads furthermore to an unpleasant inner pressure on the solar plexus. When Gaylord Hauser in his books speaks of the 'death which dwells in the bowels' he does not say enough, because such negative emotions as fear, irritability and depression also dwell there. The premature ageing of obese people is mostly caused by self-poisoning due to the sluggish functioning of their bowels.

ONE ELIMINATION A DAY IS NOT ENOUGH

Very often a patient does not realise the effect of these poisons but he proudly points out his 'regularity'. Every morning – just like clockwork – he says. An evacuation once every twenty-four hours is already a delay of twelve hours. Generally speaking, an obese person carries around the waste of about six meals. He never experiences the ideal condition of a meal passing through the digestive apparatus (like a closed parcel) and allowing the intestines to be empty and rest between meals. Westerners very rarely experience the wonderful body sensation which happens when a very good breakfast has been eaten after complete evacuation. Rejuvenation begins in the intestines.

RESTORATION OF THE ORGANS

Rejuvenation cannot be achieved through elimination of poisonous waste and irritants alone. With the regular and constant discipline of Yoga exercises, anatomical changes are brought about. Certain organs become smaller, which is often very desirable. Particularly the stomach will occupy less space, and therefore it will not press on other organs. The intestines return to their proper place. While chronic poisoning sometimes goes un-noticed, obese people are usually conscious of the weight and size of their abdomen. Obese women particularly will find their large belly a depressing disfigurement. Pressure from a flatulent stomach on the solar plexus is felt less, but is equally harmful and likely to cause depression.

INVERSION AS A REMEDY

The Yoga exercises aim at removing the cause of a heavy abdomen by reducing it to its original shape. By putting begin-ners on their shoulders and advanced students on their head, Yoga gives the inner organs a chance to return to their proper position. The undulation of abdominal breathing acts as a pneu-matic massage which speeds up the desired return of the organs to their proper places in the abdomen and simultaneously helps them to reduce their size. For fat or clumsy people who cannot achieve the Shoulderstand there are other exercises with a similar purpose. They are not as drastic but still effective, and if the student practises them for a while he will eventually gra-duate to the Shoulderstand. We must also remember that man

Biological ageing due to DISPLACEMENT WEAR POISONING NEGLECT

AGEING →

← REJUVENATION

Formerly aged becoming young again

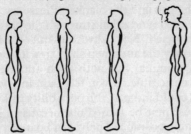

originally was a quadruped and that his body has not yet quite adapted itself to the upright position. If we are negligent about our posture in middle age, the organs will begin to sag. Only a conscious strengthening of the abdominal muscles can prevent or correct this sagging.

The inversion which is practised in Yoga postures has the effect of pushing, pressing and pulling the inner organs back into their right position. The corpulent student will be relieved to find that his lump of a stomach is actively collaborating with him. One can experience a considerable improvement only when, besides doing the exercises, one consciously 'invites' the organs to return to their proper place.

As we have seen, we can effect a state of relaxation simply by de-tensioning our facial muscles. In a similar way it is poss-ible to influence the movements of the inner organs and the flattening of the abdominal wall by a thought process, a 'listen-ing inside' and an 'inviting'.

EXERCISE: THE CONTEMPLATIVE BREATH

When you lie on your back with your knees bent and touching each other and your feet slightly apart, you invite the abdominal organs to sink back into the pelvic girdle. The back lies flat on the floor and the elbows rest on the blanket while the hands are placed on the abdomen. The breath flows calmly in and out through the nostrils.

So far, the breath was the most important thing for us. Now we go with our consciousness to the small of the back which should be lying flat like a frying pan. There is no space between the bottom of the pan and the blanket. Please try. Now breathe, relax your face, inhale and exhale through the nose; your breathing continues by itself. Not 'I breathe' but 'It breathes'. Then observe how slowly the abdomen sinks in with each exhalation. At first this is minimal but with each further exhalation it becomes more noticeable. If you feel pain in your back during this exercise, it could indicate the possibility of lordosis (hollow back). This must first be ironed out because a hollow back is a sign of a wrongly positioned pelvis and danger to your health. It is true that the human spine shows a slight S curve by nature – this has evolved as a counter-balance to our vertical posture – but this curve is only admissible if it is flexible. When the spine is stiff and immobile, a hollow back becomes dangerous.

AWAY WITH THE HOLLOW BACK

When a person develops signs of obesity, the first indication is an increase of the waistline. The second phase starts when the weight of the abdomen becomes so great that the pelvis, which is fixed to the base of the spine, tilts forward. Once this has happened the weight is mostly carried by the abdominal wall. The belly becomes shapeless and the obese person loses sight of his knees which, in future, he can see only in the mirror.

But even young and slim people can be plagued by a hollow back. This leads to the over-use of the fifth lumbar vertebra, causing lumbago and wrongly distributed weight on the feet. People who habitually stand with all their weight on one leg are also likely to acquire a hollow back.

Important precaution: The following exercises should be done preferably with an empty stomach either before breakfast or before the evening meal. A blanket should be folded double to avoid getting chilled from the floor. (It is dangerous to do these exercises on a soft or unsteady surface.) All breathing, except if indicated otherwise, must be done through the nose.

SHOULDERSTAND

There are two kinds of Shoulderstand: the straight version, called *sarva-anga-asana* in Sanskrit, and the inclined version,

FOR THE SLIM

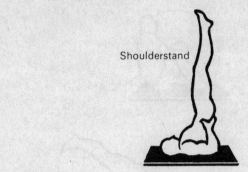

Shoulderstand

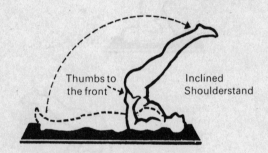

Thumbs to
the front

Inclined
Shoulderstand

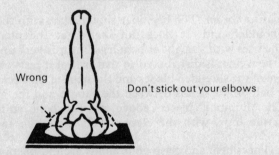

Wrong

Don't stick out your elbows

FOR THE OBESE

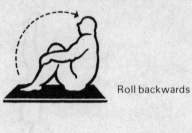

Roll backwards

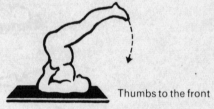

Thumbs to the front

Lower legs
and support feet
on table or back
of chair

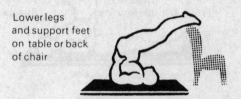

called *viparita-karani*. The beginner should start with the inclined Shoulderstand. It does not matter at the moment
whether he rises with straight or bent legs but it is very important that the weight is distributed so that half of it rests on the
upper edge of the shoulder-blades and the nape of the neck and
the other half on the hands between the thumb and the index
finger. The thumb is placed above the hip bone and the
palms on the hips, with the elbows well tucked in to the
body.

Sit with knees bent and clasp your hands around them, then
roll backwards onto your shoulders. You will find it helpful to
have a chair or a table in position on which you can rest your

feet. This will give you a feeling of security and leave you mentally free for the next step.

Exhale through the mouth — Haaa!

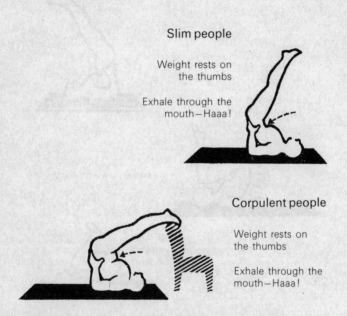

Slim people

Weight rests on
the thumbs

Exhale through the
mouth—Haaa!

Corpulent people

Weight rests on
the thumbs

Exhale through the
mouth—Haaa!

The Shoulderstand should become a rest position for you. Please keep half of your weight supported in the crook of your hands as before, otherwise it becomes exhausting and the abdominal wall remains tense although it must be sufficiently relaxed for breathing. Now, still in the same position, inhale and exhale. Inhale through the nose. Exhale 'haaa' through the open mouth. This 'haaa' should come from the depth of your chest, not as a quiet but a very clear 'haaa' breath, you then will notice that the abdomen moves inwards. This is the massage and the replacement of the organs which were mentioned before. Perform six inhalations, six 'haaa' breaths and then roll backwards as follows:

Returning to starting pose

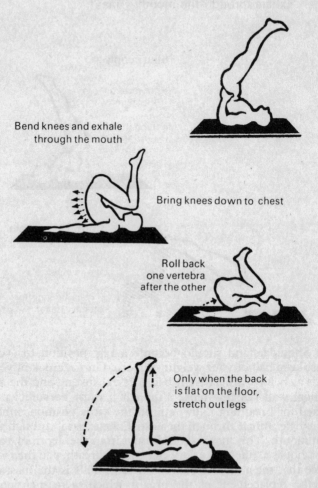

Bend knees and exhale
through the mouth

Bring knees down to chest

Roll back
one vertebra
after the other

Only when the back
is flat on the floor,
stretch out legs

AFTER THE BACKROLL COMES THE CONTEMPLATIVE
BREATH

Put a cushion under your head and place your hands on the
abdomen. Keep your knees bent. Relax your face, put the
tongue behind the lower teeth, breathe with the abdomen. Eyes
are closed; look inward. Now you will notice in which way the
exercise affected you and whether anything moves or gurgles
in your abdomen. Take six breaths, then pause and repeat the
Shoulderstand (naturally without the cushion under the head).

Precaution: It is important to remember that if you do not
hold these pauses you are not doing Yoga. Beginners should
not repeat the Shoulderstand more than five times. People with
hernia, lesions, large operational scars as well as disc trouble
in the lumbar region, must ask the doctor before beginning
these exercises.

When rolling back, the vertebrae should come onto the floor
one after the other. This is the 'ironing out' of a hollow back.
It is possible that one gets a little pain in the back; however,
should there be a strong pain, it is advisable to find out whether
you have any disc trouble in the lumbar region. Similar defects
in the region of shoulders or nape of the neck are no obstacle
to the Shoulderstand, but could prove difficult for the headstand.

The drawing up of both knees simultaneously intensifies the
pull of gravity considerably, the stomach is compressed and
moves back to its original place. For this, the solar plexus is
grateful and rewards the student with an intensified development of warmth during the subsequent Contemplative Breath.

The most important effect of this exercise is the 'sinking in'
of the abdomen, the pulling out and pushing of the intestines
from their position in the pelvis, the compression during
exhalation and the expansion during inhalation. Every exhalation achieves a deep curving of the diaphragm up into
the thoracic space, resulting in a massage of the lungs. If a
student starts coughing during this exercise it shows that he
needs it.

The plump and the weak are incapable of performing the
Shoulderstand at the beginning. For them we will substitute

another exercise. If the weakness and obesity is not caused by injury or old age, it should be remedied by cure and correction.

A plump person will find even the simplest exercise somewhat strenuous and he should therefore try to empty the bowels and reduce his body fluids with the help of fasting, sauna and special herbal teas which act on the kidneys. Naturally the exercises will be a great deal more effective if done in combination with a regime to lose weight.

FOR THE OBESE AND WEAK

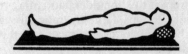

Lying on the back

Most corpulent people have round shoulders and a hollow back, hence the cushion

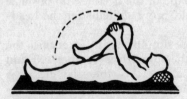

Clasp hands round the knees and exhale through the mouth

Always start with the right leg; alternately bend the leg and then relax it.
Three times each, right and left leg

The exercise described above acts as a massage of the abdomen. After a few days or weeks of practising the abdomen becomes more elastic. The pressure of the chin against the chest, intensified by the use of a pillow, acts on the thyroid. As this mostly is underactive in fat people, it helps to raise the metabolism. Furthermore, if breathing becomes easier, the student notices that his posture has improved. Even before losing any weight, one's skirts and trousers become looser around the waist.

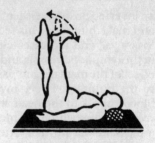

Foot circling:
Bend toes forwards then backwards
Roll feet in both directions
Slowly lower straight legs

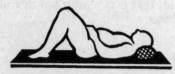

Contemplative Breath
Breathe through nose

The back as flat as a frying pan

FOOT EXERCISES ARE GOOD FOR EVERYBODY

According to Indian opinion, man ages first in the pituitary and in the ankles. With ageing the pituitary, as the conductor of the whole orchestra of the glandular system, produces disorder and disharmony in their functions. The ankles get stiff and the circulation of lymph and blood is obstructed. There are even young people who begin to show signs of this premature ageing.

This stiffening can have various causes. In the obese it is the result of overweight, as the body's structure is only calculated to carry a certain weight. If this is exceeded, a shifting of the pelvis and alteration in the bone structure of the feet (such as flat feet) are caused.

Slim people, too, can be affected by premature ageing of the ankles, it can be caused by various things such as wrong shoes, high heels or a lack of use of their feet. People who spend a great deal of time in cars pay far more attention to them than to their own bodies, of which they only think seriously when their hearts begin to protest.

An Indian doctor may immediately put his heart patient into

an inverted posture, either the Shoulderstand or the Headstand, and make him circle his feet. This practice massages the slack 'passages' and increases circulation. It prevents the stoppage in the lymphatic vessels and the veins, partly through the direct effect of the massage and partly through the richer blood supply to the pituitary. Every inversion of posture means increased blood supply to the head and to the whole body. This is easily recognised when one comes up after the Headstand and feels a pleasant warmth pervade the whole body.

Circling the feet, while in an inverted posture, is important in stimulating normal circulation. To put it in a nutshell: the feet are warm once more. This in itself is such a relief and blessing for many people, fat or thin, that it is almost worthwhile practising Yoga to have warm feet.

CIRCLING THE FEET IN THE SHOULDERSTAND

Both slim and obese people are advised to practise the Shoulderstand and to circle their feet, alternatively bending both knees while holding this posture. It is, however, essential to point out one possible danger of which every student should be conscious.

Precaution: People with overactive thyroid and similar symptoms are strongly advised not to practise the Shoulderstand; if they should attempt it they must make absolutely sure not to press the chin against the chest. If any pressure is felt, this exercise *must* be omitted.

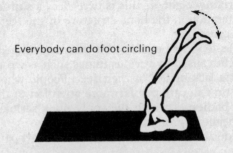

Everybody can do foot circling

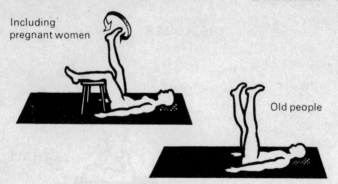

Including pregnant women

Old people

SHOULDERSTAND (SARVA-ANGA-ASANA OR THE CANDLE)

The Candle is the upright Shoulderstand which should only be practised by an obese person if he is sure that he would not fall backwards. In this posture the hands do not support the hipbone but the back of the rib cage so that the whole trunk is upright. There are variations of the foot rolling during this exercise such as: both feet circling clockwise or both feet circling anti-clockwise or both feet circling in opposite directions inwards or both feet circling in opposite directions outwards. (This can also be practised with each foot separately.) During this practice it is essential to keep the legs still.

Sarva-anga-asana is usually followed by *hala-asana* (Plough). Lowering the hips slightly, the arms are stretched out parallel with the body. Do not force the feet down to the floor or strain but exhale with the 'haaa' breath (mouth open) and go down as far as you can with straight legs. At the beginning it is advisable to place a pile of books behind your head on which to rest your toes. Remove one book each week until your feet finally touch the floor. For fat or weak people a stool or the back of a heavy chair should be used at the beginning to rest the feet upon. Try to remain in this posture for 10 to 15 seconds and then return as described on page 62. Exhale with 'haaa' and follow this by Contemplative Breathing.

THE PLOUGH

For the slim

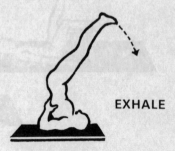

EXHALE

Hold for 15 seconds with
shallow breathing

Remove one book each week

For the corpulent

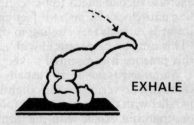

EXHALE

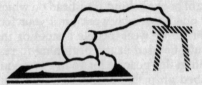

Stool or Chair

Precaution: If the Plough causes sciatic pain it should not be practised. The effect of the Shoulderstand combined with the Plough is very strong. The intestines are pressed against the diaphragm, and they are massaged and squeezed together. The re-positioning of the inner organs is strongly promoted and can be felt and experienced during Contemplative Breathing.

CHINLOCK

The Shoulderstand, and to even a stronger degree the Plough, effect a pressure of the chin against the sternum. This is a conscious stimulation of the thyroid which, in obese and phlegmatic people, usually is under-functioning. Normal people, too, find it helpful. One should watch and find which causes the better reaction: the pressure from the chin down or the chest upwards.

IMPORTANT!

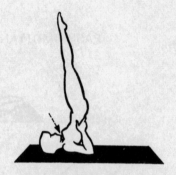

Important: For certain women (rarely for men) the chinlock has a bad effect. Those with swollen thyroids, must, under no circumstances, use it, but it is possible and even advisable to practise *viparita-karani*, as one can avoid any kind of pressure on the throat during this posture. In such cases one also uses the exercise less often and for a shorter time. However, sometimes it can be recommended to do the Headstand straight away. During periods and after the third month of pregnancy inverted postures should be discontinued.

FORWARD BENDING (PASHCIMOTTANA-ASANA)

The efficacy of the Shoulderstand and the Plough can be increased when, after having returned to the prone posture, the arms are stretched over the head so that they lie flat on the floor. Then exhale 'haaa' and, quickly bending forward, catch the big toes; the hamstrings are flat on the floor. Move the head up and down to the knees several times. Inhale deeply and roll back, arms high over the head, and exhale slowly through the nose; draw up the knees (soles of feet on the floor) and begin with Contemplative Breathing.

Important: In this case the 'haaa' exhalation must be done slowly and soundlessly. Now join these two exercises as follows: *Viparita-karani* – six times 'haaa' exhalation – Plough – rolling back – Forward Stretch – rolling back – Contemplative Breath.

Shoulderstand – foot exercises – Plough – rolling back – Forward Stretch – rolling back – Contemplative Breath.

PASHCIMOTTANA

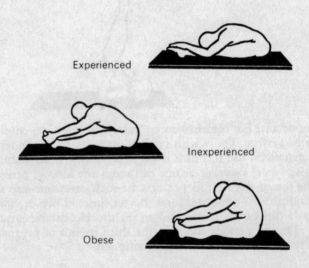

Experienced

Inexperienced

Obese

TAKE CARE OF YOUR SPINE

Do not strain forward further than you can comfortably go. A slight pain under the thighs and knees can be expected at first. The obese should try to do their best and they will surely improve in time. Forward bending can also be practised while standing, although it is more difficult.

MORNING STIFFNESS

Everybody is stiffer in the morning than in the evening. Some people find it very difficult to practise their postures before breakfast. If you really find it impossible then practise at any other time of the day as long as your stomach is empty. There are ways and means of loosening the morning stiffness, either by performing the swinging exercises described in this chapter or by practising the Contemplative Breath while still in bed, to relax back, shoulders and abdomen. Better still, do both.

THE CONTEMPLATIVE BREATH BEFORE GETTING UP

Contemplative Breathing practised when still in bed with drawn-up knees, is a conscious relaxation. Many people sleep with partly tensed muscles; in many cases they clench their fists and grind their teeth and even contract their scalp. Yoga teaches that when waking up one should smile and inhale deeply and immediately go into the posture and create the inner collected-ness of the Contemplative Breath. Begin to practise this every morning and continue with it until it has become a habit. Begin with a slow 'breath wave' and contemplation. This is followed by the invitation of warmth and repositioning of the intestines. The warmth thus created relaxes the muscles and sinews of back and pelvis. Notice the relaxation of the scalp and the way in which your problems are, as it were, carried away with each exhalation.

To the observance of movements in the intestines with the usual gurgling and flowing of the digestive juices, we now add a new form of 'invitation': the contemplation of the movements of digested food and by learning to become aware and feel its temporary resting place. Usually this internal awareness of the movement of the digestive apparatus comes only with experience, but occasionally even beginners have this gift (without realising it). This means that one can 'invite' yesterday's evening meal to move on from the small to the large intestines. You can learn to experience and direct the slow forward-creeping movements of the peristalsis. This mental direction is very useful in the achievement of 'elimination at will'. It is an essential element of Hatha-Yoga which, without this mental awareness and direction, would be difficult to tell apart from the teachings of any other physical exercises in the West.

AID TO SELF-CORRECTION

This morning introspection leads to new discoveries as one becomes familiar with one's body. Sometimes it may complain 'those fried potatoes last night gave me a lot of trouble, today things are much worse than the day before yesterday when we only had apples to digest. And these contractions in the intestines! You shouldn't pour such a lot of cold stuff into me, I am constantly on the defence!'

When you notice how this introspection functions and, particularly, when you remember the SOS signals of your body, then you begin to change your habits by switching over to active self-help. The natural change in your eating habits will come automatically from your own instinct and not because a teacher or a textbook told you to cut out certain foods. This is why the Indians say, 'do your exercises and then you'll see'.

There could be no better proof for the obese than the experience of elimination when getting up after the daily morning 'introspection'. After his exercises there could even be a second elimination and half an hour later a third. This experience will teach him to use a different yardstick for the pleasures of his palate; he will discover that he prefers this heavenly warmth in the solar plexus to a second slice of an excellent cake. This is active self-control.

In connection with elimination at will, yet another word about an important 'trick'. If after a certain exercise you have produced an elimination, you should do the Contemplative

Breath for approximately half a minute and then repeat the same exercise several times. This, presumably, will be followed by another elimination. You will also learn to judge how much food and drink and of what kind your body can take; in other words 'know thyself'.

STRETCHING AND SWINGING FOR LOOSENING UP

This and the following exercises belong to the group of tri-kona-asana (three-cornered posture). They can be executed by everybody although with different degrees of perfection. The first exercise is done standing with legs apart.

THE WINDMILL

In this exercise you stretch up as if wanting to touch the ceiling. The arms are stretched out throughout and their movement should resemble that of the arms of a windmill. It is essential to focus exactly behind you on the wall and to look at it every time you twist backwards. The feet stand parallel on the floor and the body swings once to the right and once to the left, i.e. once backwards and once forwards.

UP AND DOWNWARDS SWING

Stand with legs apart. Link your hands and inhale while stretching up. Twist the trunk to the right, bend down and touch the right foot, exhaling. Swing to the left foot and rise up to the left, inhaling. Return to the centre. The knees are kept straight throughout.

TRIANGULAR POSTURE

Stand straight with legs apart and arms stretched out sideways. Bring the right shoulder slightly forward. Twist the trunk to the left and exhale while bending down to the left foot; touch the heel with the hand and look upwards; lean back whilst you straighten up and start inhaling. The left hand glides along the calf and the right hand is stretched. This *trikona-asana* or Tri-

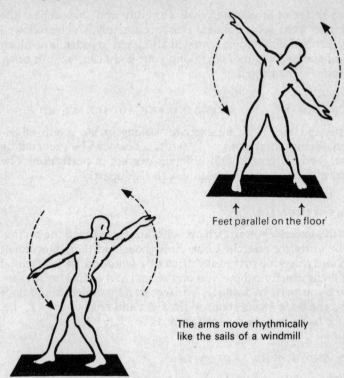

Feet parallel on the floor

The arms move rhythmically like the sails of a windmill

angular posture involves a sideways bending of the trunk which brings forward the opposite shoulder to the side you are bending. It is essential to lean slightly back when rising and to draw the hand up the back of the calf, and also to lean backwards while inhaling.

All these exercises should be repeated three times to each side.

To sum up: So far we have gone through two breathing exercises, three loosening-up exercises and those in the prone position. The last group also includes the Contemplative Breath which is always repeated between the *asanas*. The reader will

Up and Downwards Swing

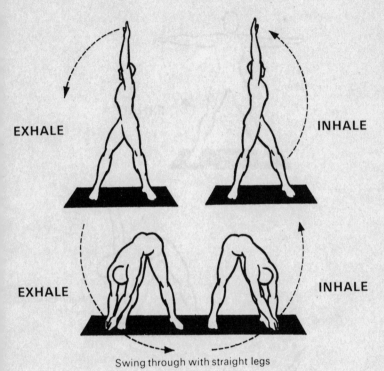

EXHALE

INHALE

EXHALE

INHALE

Swing through with straight legs

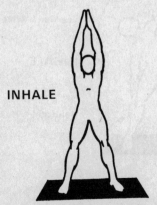

INHALE

Trikon-Asana (Triangular Posture)

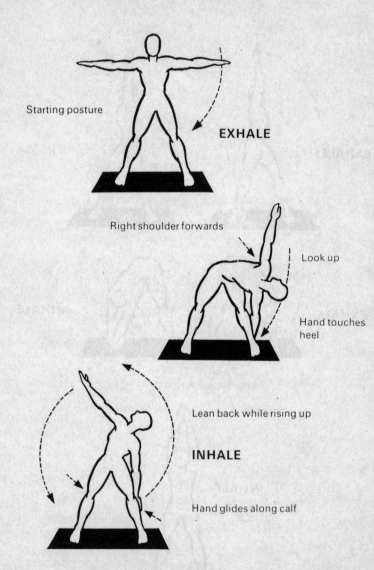

Starting posture

EXHALE

Right shoulder forwards

Look up

Hand touches heel

Lean back while rising up

INHALE

Hand glides along calf

THE SEQUENCE OF THE EXERCISES

Exercise	Name and Description	Number of repetitions	Mental Focus
Breathing	(a) *Bhastrika* in the Thunderbolt posture or on chair.	6 l./6 r.	Cleansing of nasal passages
	(b) Complete Breathing in the Thunderbolt posture or on chair.	6	Tranquillity
Loosening	(a) Windmill	6	Loosening of shoulders
	(b) Up and downwards swing	6	Freedom of movement
	(c) Triangular posture	3 each side	Stretching of the hips
Asanas	(a) Contemplative Breath in the prone position		Contemplation
	(b) *Viparita-karani* 6 times 'haaa' breath, rolling back, Contemplative Breath.	2	Abdomen
	(c) *Viparita-karani* 6 times 'haaa' breath, foot circling, Plough rolling back, Contemplative Breath	1	Abdomen and solar plexus
	(d) Shoulderstand foot rolling, Plough, rolling back, Forward Stretch, rolling back, Contemplative Breath	1	Solar plexus
	For the weak and obese, Prone position, drawing up of the knees, 3 times left, 3 times right, foot circling	6	Abdomen
		6	

ask how to include these and further exercises in a programme lasting only for 20 minutes. First of all – no hurry. The two breathing exercises must be done very calmly and be followed by the *bhastrika* breath which takes approximately 1 minute, while the following Complete Breathing takes another $1\frac{1}{2}$ minutes (six breaths), that is altogether $2\frac{1}{2}$ minutes.

The loosening-up exercises also should not be done in a hurry but in a quiet flow, for about $1\frac{1}{2}$ minutes altogether. The Shoulderstand, performed three times with $\frac{1}{2}$ minute each of the Contemplative Breath in between, will take about 6 minutes, later a little less. This means that we have now reached a programme of about 10 minutes. The further ten minutes will be dedicated to the remaining exercises.

Important: It is essential to practise the exercises in the indicated order and with a mental attitude of peace and collectedness. No hurry. If you take a little longer it does not matter.

Before going any further it is necessary to give more details on the subject of digestion as the exercises will prove more beneficial when you are fully aware of the functioning of the whole digestive system.

IV

Nutrition and Wellbeing

THE FORGOTTEN INSTINCT

It is amazing to what extent we in the West have forgotten our natural instincts. Sometimes it takes us a long time to realise that our gall bladder is sensitive to fats or that too much salt will affect us in other undesirable ways. The student of Hatha-Yoga, practising the preceding exercises regularly will, after some time, find that he is recovering his lost instincts. He will quickly discover what is good and what is bad for him.

A meal is easily digested when it is well chewed and eaten in a peaceful frame of mind, not distracted by worries or over-stimulated by reading. It is well known that the mental attitude can influence the digestion of food to a considerable extent. In India a teacher will not preach and demand moderation and restraint in the matter of food because he knows that in due course the student will choose the right foods by himself.

TRUE AND FALSE RHYTHM

Many people suffer all their lives from a false rhythm. This only becomes apparent when it is compared with the true rhythm. Ideally, nutrition and elimination happen in an eight-hour cycle. This means that preferably the evening meal has been digested and eliminated before breakfast on the following morning. The breakfast should leave the body during the after-noon and lunch ought to be eliminated before bedtime. A person who masters this ideal rhythm allows half of his digestive apparatus to rest, since when the stomach is active, large tracts of the intestines will be empty and therefore resting, which enables them to contract tightly. The digestive pulp of each meal passes through at one go and leaves no residue. This means that somebody who adopts this rhythm frees himself from waste and toxins.

It is natural that a Raja-Yogi, with his vegetarian food, frequent fasts and only two meals a day, constantly experiences this rhythm and considers it an essential. For a Westerner who cannot and would not live on 100 grams of rice a day, this is only of theoretical interest. What is important for him is the fact that there are many positive-thinking people in India who are able to realise the same rhythm without living on the simplest of diets. These are usually members of the upper classes, The kshatriyas and the intelligentsia, who employ the best cooks in the country and yet, with three to four excellent meals a day, manage to keep the ideal rhythm all their lives. They have timeless faces and youthful bodies, even in old age. One cannot judge whether they are 38 or 65 years old, but unfortunately there are not many people who have a chance of realising this. Western doctors have no contact with these people as they are never ill, nor are they likely to write books about their way of life, and therefore doctors often refuse to believe these facts.

The secret of a long life and of lifelong youthfulness lies to a great extent in the mastery of elimination. For the Western doctor the voluntary control of the peristaltic movement is often unimaginable, as is the conscious emptying of the gall bladder and the influence on the activity of the kidneys, which all depend upon the autonomic nervous system. Seen in this light, one of the traditional Indian stories is quite feasible: It describes how a ruler fathered an heir and went into battle the next day, where he was killed. This happened on his 99th birthday.

This mastery of the body can only be achieved when, from youth onwards, people have become accustomed to the emptying of stomach and bowels and never ceased practising Yoga. For the Western 20-minute Yogi, with his dilated and displaced organs, it means great progress when he manages the twelve-hour cycle. He will thus be able to rejuvenate himself at least to a certain extent. Perhaps once during a long holiday he will

The overloading of the system shown as a graph

It is expressed by the curve and shows how the overloading happens with two or more meals. The arrow indicates elimination.

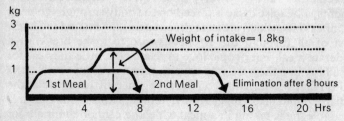

Ideal Rhythm

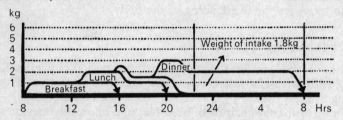

False Rhythm
Elimination after 24 hours and longer

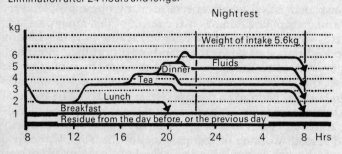

Note: For the sake of simplification, liquids and solids are considered together as if they were mixed in the bowels. The overlapping of time of two meals in the body is represented by the upper curve. The arrow indicates elimination.

be able to experience the eight-hour cycle for a short time with the help of rest, fasting and moderation. This will be an unforgettable period of his life, and he will emerge as a different person.

Even the normal twelve-hour cycle brings consistent benefits. The false cycle is forced on the body through ignoring the inner voice which indicates 'too much – too fat and too late'; most of all through the erroneous idea to make breakfast a moderate meal. Fat people love to relate how little they eat for breakfast, but they are reluctant to mention their lunch. It is natural that Western man, who works generally harder than the Indian, should take a bigger lunch; although this is quite understandable, he is taking in a meal which he cannot eliminate for at least eighteen hours. A late and heavy meal in the evening also increases the overloading of the body.

OVERLOADING AT BEDTIME

The false cycle makes the night an habitual period of overloading with the highest demands on the digestive apparatus. The sluggishness caused by overeating is increased by a person reclining in an easy chair or in bed. The pile-up in the intestines of three to five digested meals acts as a pressure on the solar plexus from within. According to Indian opinion the well-known depression which affects so many obese people every morning at about 4.00 a.m., is the result of this inner pressure.

It is strange that so few Westerners realise how this nightly overloading begins slowly to expand and distort their intestines. They are not stretching evenly like a thin tube becoming a wide tube, but rather the tube becoming a string of wide pockets separated by contracted passages. (See page 20.) The constant residue in these pockets contaminates the freshly digested matter and causes gases to develop. Compare this with the elasticity and smooth working of the intestines of the Yogi whose food passes through smoothly and quickly. For a constipated person evacuation is a constant battle. All the food has to pass from pocket to pocket through ring-like contractions. All too often he gives up the battle and takes to laxatives which act violently on the cramped intestines. It is only possible to achieve a per-

manent cure if the constipated and particularly the obese decide
not only to eat less but also to change their habits. Once it has
been understood how absolutely essential this is, they will also
find the necessary strength to keep up the essential disciplines.

It is not easy to break a false cycle, for it is usually firmly
implanted by habit and has become part of the obese's whole
life style. He now has to decide which way he would prefer:
The choice is his and the measures can be mild, energetic or
drastic.

PRACTICAL ADVICE

For the physically afflicted, cardiac patients or old and weak
people, only the mildest measures can be applied. They should
first go on a diet under medical supervision in order to lose as
much of the excess body fluid as possible. Only during the
second half of the cure should the exercises intended for this
particular type of patient be taken up and as a result the inner
massage and shrinking of the pockets will start. Furthermore,
some special exercises for this group will be described. Obese
men and women who are from four to sixteen kilos ($9\frac{1}{2}$–30 lb)
overweight should start replacing their evening meal with fruit
at least once or possibly several times a week. A fruit meal is
not like fasting as the fruit cleanses the intestines and removes
the residue. It can consist of fresh or dried fruit such as prunes,
figs or raisins (with stones). Dried fruit should only be taken
in small quantities. A good plate of salad is also permissible,
prepared in a palatable way with oil, for instance. This salad
should not include cabbage, root vegetables or potatoes. Then,
later on before going to bed, a carton of yoghourt is permitted.
If they do not like fruit they can just have the salad and yoghourt. If they can manage it, they ought to stick to this evening
meal for a week or even a whole month. The fruit will remove
the overburdening of the body and stimulate the appetite for
breakfast.

For a proper breakfast they can have an egg, porridge and
some fruit, and drink coffee or tea or whatever is preferred.
With this the false cycle can be broken. All of a sudden it will
be easy to eat less for lunch and in the evening to have again

only fruit. In the morning, a quarter of an hour after getting up, they should drink a glass of warm water, then go back to bed and practise the Contemplative Breathing, listening to the sounds in the abdomen and trying to learn what their body wants to tell them; then they should get up and start with the exercises.

Important: People who suffer from wind are always inclined to permanently control it by contraction and retention. This control should be consciously released during the Contemplative Breathing. They should lie with the knees drawn up before going to sleep, practising deep breathing and relaxation. Lying on the side with one knee up and changing sides from time to time is also advisable. All these are first steps for the necessary process of detoxication.

OVERLOADING WITH FLUID

There is yet another kind of overloading which often occurs among obese people. It is not a retention of firm residue but of fluid. The liquid swells the spongy tissues, not because the intestines are stretched but because the kidneys cannot filter the liquid fast enough. Yoga offers effective help for people with this complaint. There are first of all the *asanas* performed lying on the abdomen which massage and stimulate the kidneys; there is also the direction of warmth and concentration on one's inside to help the lazy kidneys. This works for everybody, slim or corpulent alike.

V

Exercises Lying on the Abdomen

SOME HINTS

The following exercises are called the Cobra, the Locust and the Bow. The Cobra can be attempted by every student including the uncoordinated. The Locust in its classical form would present difficulties for them, therefore they are introduced to an easier version. The Bow can only be attempted by those with a supple body.

Important: People with hernias, operational scars on the abdomen or thorax must watch their reaction to these exercises, and they should first ask their doctor whether they could undertake them. People with an overactive thyroid should omit back-bending exercises.

THE COBRA (BHUJANGA-ASANA)

Some beginners might find this exercise difficult, particularly when they are told to look up. The exercise affects the abdominal organs very strongly and acts as a massage on the kidneys. It often happens that urination is considerably increased when obese people start with the Cobra.

Uncoordinated people will find the exercise strenuous but as it only uses the back muscles, the heart is not strained and it can therefore be attempted by the weak as well.

After two repetitions of the Cobra practise the Contemplative

THE SLIM	THE OBESE
INHALE	Lift the abdomen

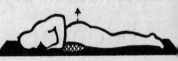

1. Abdominal breathing

Bend head back   Hold the breath

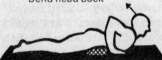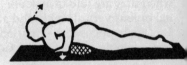

2. Lift trunk
   No pressure on the hands
   Weight rests on the pillow

3. Up to here no weight on the hands

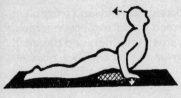 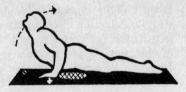

4. Take the weight on the hands
   Raise the abdomen only ½ inch
   Do not do press-ups
   Hold the breath
   Allow the body to descend

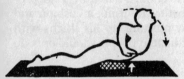 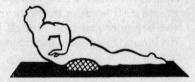

5. Exhale through the mouth: Haaa!
   Rest the abdomen on the cushion
   Raise the hands and slowly sink back

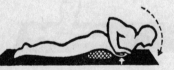 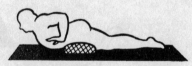

6. Continue to sink back
   The cushion massages the abdomen

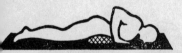 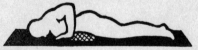

7. Lower forehead
   Breathe shallowly

   Repeat the whole 3 times

Breath. This is especially important for old and corpulent people. A feeling of cold may disturb the introspection which, in this case, is directed mainly towards the kidneys and the small of the back. It is advisable to cover the legs with a blanket. Imagine the small of the back as a frying pan getting slowly warm on the stove. Feel the warmth beginning to spread to the kidneys and the whole of this region. Imagine that the kidneys absorb the warmth as if they were sponges; feel them expand, basking in this comfortable warmth.

THE LOCUST (SHALABHA-ASANA)

This is the most strenuous exercise of our 20-minute Yoga programme. It is easier to do this posture by using a cushion and the beginner can help himself by pushing up his thighs with his hands. Corpulent and uncoordinated people should only do

ACROBATICS ARE NOT A SIGN OF THE TRUE YOGI

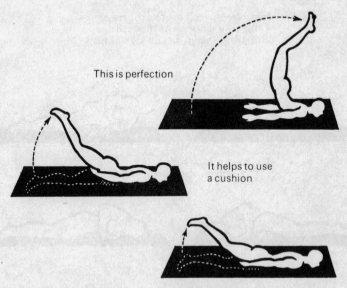

This is perfection

It helps to use
a cushion

Daily practice is the sign of sincerity

THE SLIM   THE OBESE AND CLUMSY

INHALE

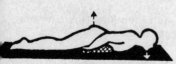

1. Raise abdomen, inhale
   Press on chin and toes
   Leave the chin on the blanket

Raise both legs   Raise one leg

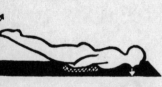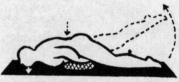

2. Hold the breath
   Legs straight
   Support the hip bone

Hold

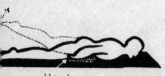

Hand

3 Slim : hold 2-4 seconds
   Obese : Exhale, release

Slowly lower legs   **EXHALE**   Lift the other leg

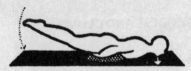 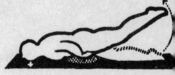

4 . Slim : Exhale through the mouth   Bring legs down straight
    Obese : Lift other leg as before

 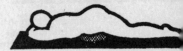

5. Both : pause
    Lie flat on the cushion
    Turn head to one side
    Take 10 shallow breaths

    Repeat the whole 3 times

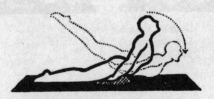

For athletes
With or without cushion
Swing up and down 6 times

half of the exercise by raising one leg at a time; relaxation
between each leg raising is necessary.

THE BOW (DHANURA-ASANA)

This exercise is not suitable for some corpulent and uncoordinated people, but it is sometimes good for fat people, especially

if they have long arms. The soft cushion is a help, but again remember to be careful if there is a history of hernia or abdominal operations. The only pain which is acceptable is the stretching pain in thighs and knees; all other kinds of pain would be a warning signal to omit this exercise.

THE CONTEMPLATIVE BREATH

Lie flat on your back, if necessary covered with a blanket. Breathe into your abdomen and observe the cold and warm flow

THE SLIM	THE OBESE

INHALE

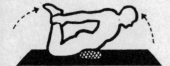 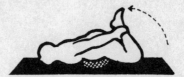

1. Inhale abdominally. Hold ankles or feet and lift

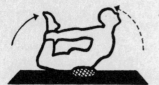 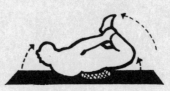

2. Hold the breath. Raise knees, thighs and head

EXHALE

3. Exhale. Relax

Repeat the whole 3 times
Then lie on your back and perform the Contemplative Breath

of your breath. Then direct your attention to the solar plexus, framed with your hands. Imagine how your back begins to warm up and how this warmth pulsates through your kidneys. Then feel how it spreads over the entire back.

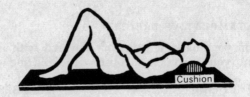

VI

Yoga for Back Trouble

IS DISC TROUBLE A DISEASE OF CIVILISATION?

I cannot believe this. I think that Western man of today has acquired all the comforts of our age but his greatest mistake is that he does not realise the dangers and consequences of spoiling himself. He is not yet civilised enough to understand the most complex of all machinery – his own body and mind. As we have chairs and tables, hardly anybody works squatting. Since water is brought into most homes, women do not carry heavy jugs on the crown of their heads from the well to their houses. The lift is in widespread use and even in those houses where there is no lift, people rarely carry boxes and baskets on their backs going upstairs. Even our porters do not live up to their name: they no longer carry the luggage themselves but use a vehicle to transport it.

Altogether we are rather pleased with our technical achievements which make life easier. Where we are mistaken is that we think that our pelvis, spine, muscles, joints, bones and sinews which are built for pressure, stretching, twisting and carrying, can function entirely without all these activities. Girls and young women should carry something on the crown of their head for several minutes each day; they should also bend and squat to keep back and pelvis in good condition. Men should lift and press down, bend and turn and tense the body, even if it is only for some minutes each day. Most of all we have to counteract one-sided stress by compensating with movements in the opposite direction.

In certain working conditions and professions, back trouble is considered a professional hazard. Right-handed dentists stand next to the chair with constant turning to the left. Long-distance drivers on lorries become a victim of non-stop vibrations. They fill the waiting-rooms of osteopaths, orthopaedic surgeons and chiropractitioners. They have neither learnt to sit properly and to relax nor how to counteract contortional stress. They face their suffering with the same helplessness with which a Papuan faces malaria. All these people are the victims of insufficient education. Prevention of their troubles can largely be learnt. Even when back trouble has already developed, Yoga can be very helpful.

ACQUIRED SPINAL DAMAGE

Congenital malformation of the spine and disturbed spinal development in children belong to a textbook of orthopaedics. On the other hand the many changes of the spine which are acquired by adolescents and grown-ups should be mentioned in a book on Yoga. To these belong the innumerable cases of displaced vertebrae which are caused by accidents and 'harmless' falls which happen so often to cyclists, skiers and particularly motor cyclists as well as horse riders. Many accidents are also caused by the wrong lifting of heavy weights.

Displacement of vertebrae either singly or in pairs is a common complaint. This is noticeable even to the layman. Put somebody on his abdomen and examine his spine with two fingers. You will notice the zig-zag position of the vertebrae. Some people cannot turn the head fully to one side, others feel pain from shoulder to fingertip. A great number of Westerners cannot stand without pain for any length of time and always are conscious of an unpleasant sensation in the small of the back.

A tilted pelvis, for instance, develops in the following way: The lowest lumbar vertebra has twisted and lies at an angle on the pelvis, pressing down on the disc and separating it from the pelvis, in bad cases down to the bone. This condition can also be caused by a twisting of other lumbar vertebrae. The tilt of the pelvis and therefore the seeming unevenness of the length of the legs go mostly undetected. They are often only noticed when the tailor has to lengthen one trouser leg. This condition deteriorates with the years if the tilt has not been corrected.

In pregnant women this tilt is often connected with an exaggeratedly hollow back. It is reasonable to assume that there is a connection between the tilted pelvis and the simultaneous formation of varicose veins. In bad cases it can even cause a complication during birth and there is far greater danger of thrombosis than with a pelvis in its normal position.

A tilted pelvis is particularly noticeable in the headstand, even when it does not show otherwise. It is quite simple to check oneself with the help of another person: Lying flat on the back, the legs are stretched out loosely with heels touching and toes slightly pointing outwards. The other person will see if one heel is lower. After a piece of paper has been placed under both heels, the checker takes a pencil and puts it upright on the paper. He then can mark on the paper the position of the heels. It is always useful to show this to a student so that he sees for himself what causes his pain.

FIRST REPLACE, THEN PRACTISE YOGA

Wherever such malformation of the spine occurs, one should not (with two exceptions) try to correct them oneself, but take professional advice. With the two exceptions which will be mentioned later, Yoga does not act as a chiropractic correction but is merely intended as a decisive help for the regeneration of a damaged spine and its restoration to full mobility. The exercises can remedy lordosis by stretching and straightening the spine, and they strengthen the ligaments so that the repositioned vertebrae cannot slip out as easily as before.

Warning: The following exercises are recommended with the supposition that the student will stick to the limitations recommended by a doctor. Nobody who has just had a cervical vertebra put back in its proper place should endeavour the Headstand. With a pelvis which has only recently been corrected one ought not to practise the Windmill or the Triangular position. After a few weeks these exercises are particularly suited to maintain and increase the symmetry of movement. Pregnant women must only practise exercises with the permission of their doctor and not continue with the special exercises any longer than the months of pregnancy mentioned in this book.

PREVENTIVE AND STRENGTHENING EXERCISES

The same exercises which serve as a prevention of spinal trouble can be used to regain the elasticity of the spine, lost, for instance, after an accident. They can be divided into two groups: asymmetrical exercises in which turning or swinging is executed first to the one and then to the other side, and symmetrical exercises in which the body is bent either forward or backward.

The exercises described on pages 75–7 are very suitable for gradually removing stiffness of the shoulders or the pelvic girdle. Together with the Triangle and the later mentioned Screw, they belong to the asymmetrical exercises. Both of these could mean too heavy a strain for students whose pelvis had only recently been put right. One must work slowly and carefully towards full flexibility.

Complete Breathing belongs to the group of symmetrical exercises and the Shoulderstand (see pages 61–4), particularly the rolling backwards from the Shoulderstand, is performed to counteract lordosis. Backwards and forwards bending is difficult for corpulent people or for those whose pelvis is tilted. They should also not attempt the *pashcimottana-asana*. Strengthening postures for the back are the Cobra, the Locust and the Bow. The Headstand with variations (see pages 129–32) is especially suitable for achieving a straight posture. Pressure on the crown of the head is a substitute for the carrying of water jars or other loads on the head.

DANDA

This and the following exercises belong to the two groups mentioned above.

Symmetrical	Asymmetrical
(1) *Danda* ('stick') – the Indian press-up	(4) Screw
(2) Cat Stretch	(5) Spiral
(3) Camel Ride	(6) Cow

The *danda* is extremely suitable for beginners. In India it is favoured by wrestlers, other sportsmen and soldiers. It is also taught in Yoga schools since it is a most effective correctional posture and the best training for weak backs. *Danda* is a part of the well-known cycle of movements called *surya-namaskara* or 'Obeisance to the Sun' (also 'Sun Prayer'), designed by the late Raja of Aundh. These postures are particularly recommended for women as a corrective and strengthening exercise as well as for people who do sedentary work and for tractor or long-distance drivers.

For the beginner (pregnancy up to the 4th month)
Lying on the abdomen as for the Cobra (without cushion), put the feet on the toes. The hands are as in the Cobra position, the forehead is on the floor. Inhale, hold the breath, look up and raise the trunk into the Cobra posture in one continuous quick movement until the arms are stretched and exhale again through the mouth. Then, with straight arms, go into the Triangular position with the buttocks as high up as possible; put the head between the arms and look at your abdomen. Contract the buttocks and pull the abdomen in. Stand on tiptoe, then bend the arms and return to the starting position. Do not stop

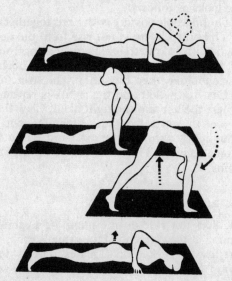

but with the next inhalation immediately assume the Cobra posture again. One execution of the *danda* needs about three seconds and should be performed in one flowing movement. How often? Middle-aged students or women should perform this exercise two to three times.

For the strong
As above, but on fingertips. First inhale, then slightly raise the abdomen one-third of an inch; only nose, head and toes touch the floor; move into the Cobra and Triangle, followed by a return to the first posture without touching the floor. During the Triangular position stand on the soles. This should be done ten to thirty times.

THE CAT STRETCH

Wild cats like a stretch in which, standing on their hind legs, they lean with their chests against a tree trunk. They try to make themselves as long as possible and hook the claws of their forelegs into the bark once to the right and once to the left. Your performance looks as follows:

Sit in the Thunderbolt posture with heels together and knees wide apart. The buttocks must not rise from the heels. Then shift the weight with a slow stretching movement from one heel to the other, bend forward and roll sideways. Touch the floor first with one shoulder, then the other. The stretching movement of the Cat – to the left and the right – is repeated several times. Alternate the left and the right hand. Claw the mat like a cat. The stretch starts from the hips. Do not bend the arms. Breathe lightly through the nose and repeat the whole for ten to fifteen seconds. This exercise often brings alleviation of sciatic pains.

THE CAMEL RIDE

In India one does not ride on the hump of a camel but in a saddle behind it, at the very end of the camel's back, and therefore one gets heavily shaken up. This exercise is done in the following way: Sit in the Thunderbolt posture with knees

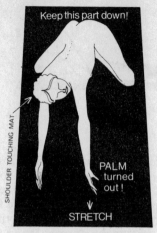

CAT STRETCH!

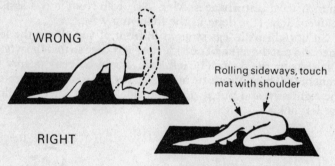

together. At the beginning it helps to put a firm cushion under both feet (not under the knees). Rise from the knees and arch backwards with body and head. Hold the insteps and heels. Bend the arms and try to produce a slightly swinging movement backwards. Do this for a few seconds and follow it with the Cat Stretch. Pregnant women should ask their doctor if and for how long they could perform these two exercises.

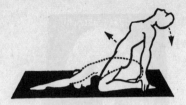

THE SCREW

In this posture the pelvis is fixed by the crossing of the arms and legs. Turn your head backwards very slowly. This movement should gradually affect the entire spine like the turning of a screw. The greatest effect is on the five lumbar vertebrae in the lower part of the back which, unlike the thoracic vertebrae, are not supported by the rib cage. Between these vertebrae issue those groups of nerves which supply the kidneys and the sexual organs, therefore this exercise has a beneficial influence on menstrual disturbances. Men also profit from it as it assists rejuvenation. It is done in the following way:

Sit upright with legs straight in front of you. Bend the left knee and put the left foot outside the right knee so that the whole sole rests on the floor. The left knee should be bent steeply in front of the chest. While turning from the hip to the left, stretch the right arm and put it down outside the left knee, holding the left ankle.

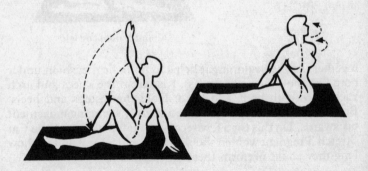

Now, with exhalation through the nose, slowly turn your head and eyes backwards to the left, trying to grasp the right knee with the left hand stretched around the waist from the back. Remain for a few seconds in this posture and then, with slow inhalation, return to the starting position. A variation consists in the following: The right arm goes under the left knee and the hands are joined behind the back.

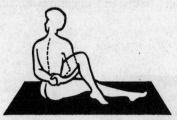

Remember: The right arm is always over the left knee and the left arm over the right knee.

Repeat this exercise once or twice, always alternating between left and right. If afterwards you feel a pleasant warmth in the lower back, the exercise has been performed correctly.

Important for women: It is advisable to perform this exercise during menstruation. If you are under orthopaedic or chiropractic treatment ask if you should do this exercise.

THE SPIRAL

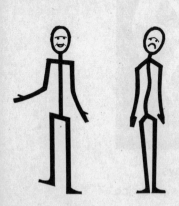

This exercise is very important, particularly for pregnant women, as it prevents after-birth thrombosis. More than half the population have a tilted pelvis and millions of older people suffer from the consequences. A tilted pelvis is recognisable by the seemingly different lengths of the legs. The displacement of two lumbar vertebrae disturbs the balance. Usually the seemingly longer leg is spared while the other is overburdened. Consequences: Back or sciatic pain, varicose veins on one side, inefficiency of the intestines particularly in pregnant women.

The Spiral corrects the displacement of the vertebrae. People with congenital damage or progressive degeneration of the spine must avoid this exercise. However, it has helped to relieve many older people from great pain and handicaps where the usual traction, massage, baths and injections failed. To help these

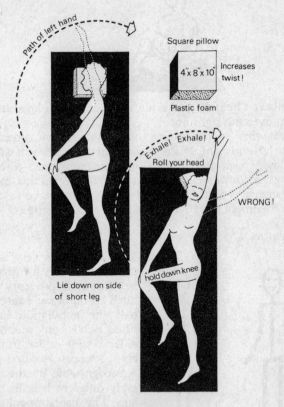

Path of left hand

Square pillow

4" x 8" x 10"   Increases twist!

Plastic foam

Exhale! Exhale!

Roll your head

WRONG!

Lie down on side of short leg

hold down knee

Do this roll both ways

– each side thrice

people with this particular exercise, the following preparation has proved efficient:

Suppose that your shorter leg is on the right side and therefore start the exercise lying on the right (important).

Take a four- to five-inch thick small cushion and lie on the right side, the right ear on the cushion and the right shoulder in front of it. (The cushion should fill the space between shoulder and ear.) Now pull up the left knee (always the upper knee) at a right angle and put it on the floor. Put both hands on that knee. The right hand holds the knee to the ground while the left hand rests lightly above it. The lower leg is stretched out relaxed. Inhale and then perform the spiral twist of the trunk during one long slow exhalation: Drag the hand over the floor and finish the twist by turning the head to the left on the cushion (rolling off the cushion increases the twist): Keep the arm over the head – stretching it for a few moments (the hand is constantly on the floor). Turn back the head and start exhaling, dragging the hand along the floor to the starting position.

No application of strength is required. No jerky movement with the arm! Repeat this two or three times, then turn over on the other side and perform the exercise in the opposite direction.

THE COW

This exercise is best done either in the Thunderbolt posture or standing. Bend the left arm, elbow up, with the hand between

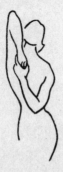

the shoulder-blades. Bend the right arm from below and try to grasp the left hand. It is possible to correct a displaced thoracic vertebra with this exercise. This is permitted auto-chiropractic. If one can do this exercise on one side and not on the other it could be caused by a displaced vertebra or a stiff wrist which prevents the reaching of the other hand.

This exercise is particularly advisable for car drivers and people who spend their time bent over a typewriter or other machines. Together with the Screw, the Spiral and the *danda* it will help to correct the one-sided posture of dentists or others who habitually use only one side in their work, or play such games as tennis or golf, etc.

VII

Yoga for Women

PREGNANT WOMEN

The important preparation for motherhood should not begin with pregnancy. Long before, a young girl must know how to deal with digestion and elimination and how to prevent colds. Years before marriage exercises should start to strengthen the back to preserve its symmetry, to correct posture and to keep the pelvis mobile. It is essential to use breathing as a source of strength and as a means of internal massage. Deep relaxation is also essential.

If all this has been omitted, everything can still be well when a young woman catches up in time with the preparation *before* her first pregnancy begins. All she has to do is a daily Yoga programme of 20 minutes in the morning which is reinforced by deep relaxation during the day.

CATCHING-UP PROGRAMME FOR YOUNG WOMEN

Type of Exercise Name / Description	Number of times	Mental Focus	Duration (seconds)
BREATHING			
A. Complete Breathing in Thunderbolt pose	6	Peace and strength	60–90
B. *Bhastrika* in Thunderbolt pose	6 left 6 right	Cleansing of sinuses	60–90 slowly

Type of Exercise Name/Description	Number of times	Mental Focus	Duration (seconds)
LOOSENING			
A. Windmill: arm swinging while standing	6 forwards 6 backwards	Loosening of the shoulders	60–90 slowly
B. Swinging through while standing with feet apart	3 left 3 right	Loosening of the pelvis	30
C. Triangular posture while standing with feet apart	3 left 3 right	Alternate stretching of hips	
D. Squatting with legs apart, soles flat, arms forward	3	Loosening of pelvis	
GENERAL STRENGTHENING			
Danda	3–6	Increasing flexibility of spine	30–60 quick
ASANAS			
I. *On the back:*			
A. Complete Breathing with bent knees	I	Concentration on centre between eyebrows	60
B. *Viparita-karani*, 6 times soundless 'haaa' breath, rolling off, Contemplative Breath (pause)	2	Abdomen	120
C. As above, with foot rolling, Plough, slow rolling forward, Forward Bending, rolling back, Contemplative Breath	2	Solar plexus	180
II. *Abdominal postures:*			
D. Cobra, pause	3	Kidney area Warmth in back	30–45 30

Type of Exercise Name/Description	Number of times	Mental Focus	Duration (seconds)
E. Locust,	3	Kidney area	30
pause		Warmth in back	30
F. Bow,	2	Kidney area	20
pause		Warmth in back	30
III. *In Thunderbolt posture:*			
G. Panther Stretch	I	Suppleness	20–30
H. Camel Ride	I	Suppleness	20
Camel Ride and Panther Stretch combined	3	Suppleness	120–150
Lying on back, with knees drawn up, Contemplative Breath	I	The centre between the eyebrows warmth in pelvis	60
IV. *Sitting with straight legs:*			
I. Twist	2 left 2 right	Alternating warmth in lower back	60
J. Contemplative Breath	I	Warmth in pelvis	60
V. *On the back:*			
K. Spiral	I left I right	Suppleness in the lower back	60
LOOSENING			
Squatting with legs apart	I	Suppleness of pelvis	60
Contemplative Breath	I		60
VI. *Headstand:*			
L. Headstand from Dolphin	I	Foot circling	30
Contemplative Breath	I	Warmth in solar plexus	60

Warning: The Abdominal Lift or *uddhiyana-bandha* (see pages 135–6) must not be attempted as soon as conception is suspected.

Under normal conditions, pregnancy exercises can be continued (in the described order) until approximately the twelfth week of pregnancy; naturally the postures must be performed particularly slowly and without any force. A doctor's advice should be sought.

YOGA AFTER THE THIRD MONTH OF PREGNANCY

In the fourth month of pregnancy the following exercises must be omitted: Shoulderstand, Plough, Forward Bending, Headstand and all exercises in the abdominal position.

LEG CRADLING (up to the fourth month)

For this exercise, which is intended to keep the pelvis elastic, sit on a blanket, bend the right knee and hold the leg with the right arm, trying to bring the foot with the sole under the left

'Rocking the Baby' for an elastic pelvis
Sit on the blanket

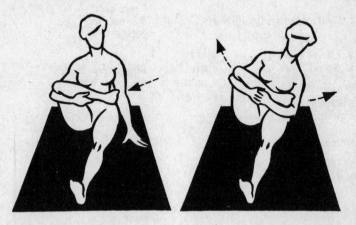

Bend the right knee

armpit. Then transfer the weight to the left buttock and link your hands lightly. Bring knee and foot to the body and perform a rocking movement from left to right. Change to the other leg and repeat. Follow this up by the Contemplative Breath lying on the back. Feel the warmth in the pelvic region (2 minutes).

In the fifth month (if not advised earlier by the doctor) omit: Danda, Windmill, Triangular posture, Camel Ride, Complete Breath in the Thunderbolt posture, Leg Cradling.

During the last months of pregnancy, if the doctor agrees, the following exercises *can* be continued: Screw (very slowly), Spiral, Foot Circling on the back. As pregnancy advances, partial and deep relaxation become more important.

LIMITATIONS OF TEACHING

Experience with several thousand Yoga beginners showed me that after several lessons a high percentage of students become aware of certain physical shortcomings which they had not suspected until then or which had been wrongly explained. This is also valid for many women who want to conceive. They discover, for instance, that they have a general weakness of the back or that a hollow back is neither normal nor desirable. Very often, this stiff hollow back is the cause of harmful complications. However, it can be corrected through Yoga. The exercises of the catching-up programme can, with certain precautions, serve to strengthen and recondition the spine to its former flexibility.

It is equally important that young women learn (with the help of the catching-up programme) how to regulate the breath and increase the capacity of the lungs, because often only a fifth or even a seventh of the full capacity is made use of. Yoga reduces the susceptibility to colds and often helps with asthma. In addition there is the psychological effect of the exercises. The pregnant woman learns the connection between the rhythm of her breath and the state of her mind and, to a certain degree, is able to master it. This is of great help when, in hours of depression, she can free herself from low spirits by deep relaxation. The breathing exercises alone lead her to the steps of contemplation and therefore to a source of comfort and peace.

There are many women who, until the sixth month of pregnancy, have never bothered to study the functions of their body. In most cases they have only tried to relieve their colds, coughs, constipation, kidney trouble, migraine etc. with tablets, pills and injections. When in the sixth month they come to the Yoga teacher with a kidney attack, varicose veins or strong pain in the back, it is too late for exercises of a dynamic kind. It is hardly possible at that stage to teach them even thoracic breathing which the well-prepared can continue with in the sixth or even seventh month. But even then they can still be taught how to relax during and after labour.

PARTIAL AND DEEP RELAXATION

The Contemplative Breath described on page 29 is a partial relaxation which can be achieved in a short time, for instance

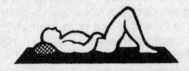

in between labour pains. Deep relaxation differs from short partial relaxation as it needs a longer preparation and excludes any movement such as a correction of the posture which would disrupt the mental collectedness. For slim people it is usually sufficient to put the legs on a cushion or mattress which also supports the heels. Pregnant women with a hollow back should put the legs from the knees downwards on an upholstered stool or couch. If even then the back does not lie flat, one can slide a cushion underneath the head to support the hollow part of the back.

Deep relaxation for the pregnant woman should take 20 to

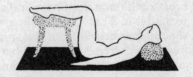

40 minutes without any change of the position and with legs and feet covered. Only under these conditions can the whole body from top to toe participate in the benefits of deep relaxation.

A BLESSING FOR MOTHER AND CHILD

This book differs from other works on Yoga particularly in one respect: It dedicates a considerable space to relaxation. For the Western reader this is especially important, for deep relaxation is the most difficult of all exercises. We are dynamically inclined and live by progressing from one task to another. To enter the sphere of non-doing and to accept a more contemplative attitude needs a good deal of effort and a certain self-discipline. The nature of deep relaxation consists in a mental attitude of non-commanding and non-interfering. It is an exercise which is not 'done' but which 'comes' by itself. The recuperation of the mind is based on this 'stepping out' from the 'aggressive' approach adopted during everyday life in which we are used to give orders and to think in terms of achieving our daily quota.

Thus, deep relaxation has not only the effect of an inner detoxication – it brings about at the same time a mental regeneration and relieves both worries and tensions. Although the psychological effects are not measurable, they can become unforgettable experiences. Deep relaxation lies at the borderline of human experience, and its possibilities are as yet only inadequately studied. Our everyday vocabulary is quite insufficient to describe the experience during deep relaxation, and new expressions have to be coined such as 'fusion' and 'step of integrity', etc. At the present stage of knowledge some of its accompanying phenomena are still completely inexplicable. Here is an example:

A middle-aged lady took several private lessons in her home. She was a healthy strong woman, several times a grandmother, well-to-do and living in her own beautiful home. But the divorce which she had to face after many years of marriage greatly depressed her. The lessons took place in a spacious room with a canary in his cage near the window. We ended each lesson with deep relaxation. The canary, who had never sung before, began to trill every time his mistress achieved complete relaxation. This happened thirteen times during thirteen lessons! It seems clear that the bird experienced the release of the woman's tensions and proclaimed his joy. How much more can the unborn child participate in the beneficial effects of its mother's deep relaxation.

YOGA AFTER BIRTH-HEALING AND RECUPERATION

Every birth leaves a wound in the mother's womb which needs time to heal. This may happen quickly – perhaps within two weeks, or it may take several months. During this period deep relaxation is most beneficial. This time it should be connected with the mental picture of a healing warmth in the womb. After this period and with the permission of her physician the mother can take up a series of special exercises aiming at replacing the inner organs and of regaining her figure.

Certain inverted postures like the Shoulderstand or variations of the Headstand will help, since they utilise the gravity which in pregnancy caused the displacement of the inner organs. During the inverted postures, while practising the soundless exhalation with completely relaxed abdominal muscles, one can feel how the organs slide back into their proper place. However, all deliberate muscular contraction should be avoided. In order to consolidate this process some of the following special exercises should be selected: Complete Breathing while kneeling, the three loosening exercises, Windmill, Swinging and the Triangular posture, *Danda*, the Shoulderstand with legs moving forward and backward and the Headstand with legs alternately stretched and bent.

For bad circulation in the legs and as a remedy for varicose veins it is advisable to circle the feet in the Shoulderstand or the Headstand; the Screw and the Spiral, left out in the catching-up programme, can now be taken up again. It is left to the intelligent observation of the individual reader to gradually expand her daily programme. To firm the breasts the following exercises are indicated: Complete Breathing, Windmill, Spiral and *Danda*. Nursing mothers hold the breasts with both hands (pillows under elbows) in deep relaxation.

This 'rejuvenation' programme of the mother through Yoga should be adopted by all post-natal clinics. Few women have an idea of how much can be achieved with it. I always remember with admiration, a princess, one of the most beautiful women of India. She was 36, had eleven children – and looked like her oldest daughter who then may have been 16 years old.

VIII

The Art of Deep Relaxation

In my experience with hundreds of students of Hatha-Yoga, half the beginners seem to achieve the sensation of warmth during the Contemplative Breath easily and quickly. It often happens even during the first few attempts, while placing the hands on the solar plexus. Others achieve this experience only after repeated attempts. Approximately a quarter of the students complain that they are unable to 'produce' the sensation of warmth. That they use the wrong approach is shown by the choice of the expression. The conscious effort of trying to 'produce' shows that the person has failed to understand the very essence of the Contemplative Breath. This wrong attitude is responsible for their failure to be passive and let go.

The conscious 'direction of warmth' is nothing but the second step of deep relaxation which follows the experience of heaviness during the first stage. This experience of heaviness can be induced in all parts of the body, for instance in the eyes, arms and legs and also in the inner organs. It is but a directed de-tensioning. It is easy to understand how to de-tense or relax if one realises how tension comes about in the first place. Linguistic usage is quite correct when it sanctions the expression that one does not 'produce' a cramp but that one 'gets' it. However, it can be removed with the technique of 'appealing to' or 'letting go'.

The Contemplative Breath is a first step in the direction of the non-doing of the Raja-Yogi. It is the beginning of every relaxation: a letting go, a passive looking on. It represents a kind of self-examination in which the harmonious interaction of body and mind is greatly enhanced.

The relaxation of an adult differs from that of a sleeping child or of an animal, as it is experienced consciously. It proceeds along the same lines and leads to the same results as the unconscious relaxation of a child but it is intensified. It is a mental process and as such the culmination of a systematic self-education: the high art of being kind to oneself.

THE EXPERIENCE OF WARMTH AS INCREASED BLOOD CIRCULATION

It is essential to realise that the experience of warmth is founded on the blood circulation throughout the body. This is only possible when the capillaries are open. Depending on their constriction or dilation, certain glands or muscles are either able or unable to function. The blood supply is subordinate to the autonomic nervous system over which we have no direct control.

This system can only be appealed to with repeated mental invitations which may have to be continued over a period of half an hour or more. It often happens that a beginner stops too soon with the Contemplative Breath. His body reacts only slowly but if he gives himself more time he will find that he, too, can achieve the experience of warmth. If the euphoric sensation of warmth does not occur after several repeated attempts, it is possible that the student has not considered the close link between body and mind.

PHYSICAL IMPEDIMENTS

The experience of warmth is in many cases prevented by the strange unkindness with which Western people treat their bodies. They flop down on the floor without considering its hardness, the cold, the draught and other factors of a similar kind. Any Indian would regard this as an incomprehensible cruelty. He would find it incredible that there are people who lie down on a blanket but leave the head to rest on a cold stone floor. He certainly would fold the blanket to protect his whole body to make himself comfortable.

The observation of such details simply belongs to the art of being kind to oneself. The sooner we adopt this oriental attitude, the further we shall go in Hatha-Yoga. It is equally natural that one should be covered with another blanket while practising the Contemplative Breath. The hands, too, should be put under the blanket. To achieve a sensation of warmth it is essential not to start with a loss of warmth. To place the hands on top of the blanket is a sure sign that the student has largely lost his bodily awareness through sheer neglect.

In one respect the Indian is apparently less sensitive than the Western student: he can endure more noise. For us it is best to practise the daily session in a period of relative quiet which presumably occurs in every household at some time or other. Besides the elimination of all disturbance, there are also positive aids. For example, one can assist circulation in the lumbar region by brushing the back in upward strokes with a strong brush before beginning with the Contemplative Breath. In India certain types of percussion and treading massages are used to assist relaxation.

MENTAL RESISTANCE

Even if all physical impediments are removed, there still remain some obstacles of a mental nature which stand in the way of deep relaxation and improved circulation. It is mainly people in an executive capacity who suffer from such complaints. It seems as if a certain resistance has been built up in their foreheads which prevents them from letting go and being passive. They also often complain to be unable to relax their foreheads. These are the victims of the well-known 'manager disease'. Their impediment is part of their whole being, for they even want to command the sensation of warmth, which of course is impossible. They live in a constant state of self-hypnosis, being driven from one activity to the next. Sometimes it happens that they burst into tears during their first relaxation.

For them it is often a great relief to discover that their bodies do not resist relaxation, but even long for it. As a matter of fact the body is only waiting for an opportunity to help itself. It is not at all necessary to give commands, for the body has known it all since birth. All it demands is that there is no interference. The relaxation with the Contemplative Breath is a kind of introspection, a passive witnessing. As such it is an introduction and a step towards the deeper meditation of Raja-Yoga. Those who have not learnt to relax will never be able to meditate.

Next to these tense and hyper-efficient people are those with a butterfly mind. They, too, are unable to feel the sensation of warmth in deep relaxation. They are too impatient to watch the performance taking place in the body. Every partial or complete relaxation is like a theatrical performance. The body is the stage, the author of the play is nature and our wakeful mind is the audience. If the audience leaves, the performance comes automatically to a stop. Hence the mind must take part in the relaxation process. This will be discussed in detail in the chapter on deep relaxation.

One of the best ways of achieving concentration is the mental observation of the movement of the breath. It is much easier to concentrate on movement than on a fixed point. It is best to get absorbed in the sensation of warmth and the regularity of the breath. In addition to this one should remember to relax the tongue as well. The rest follows. Suddenly the sensation of warmth is felt. It seems a good idea to end this section with an exercise so that all that has been said here can be put into practice right away.

Perform the Shoulderstand (*viparita-karani*) twice, then the Cobra and the Locust three times in succession and follow it with Contemplative Breathing. Relax on your back with your hands loosely framing the solar plexus. Focus your inner vision on the spot behind your eyes and observe the flow of cold and warm breath. Inhale and exhale regularly. Inhalation is cold, exhalation is warm. Visualise how the warmth is soaked up by your back and then direct your attention again to the rhythm of your breathing.

IX

Headstands

WHY THE HEADSTAND AT ALL?

The classical literature and tradition of Yoga counts the Headstand among the so-called meditational postures. The texts
demand that the Yogi remain in this posture for about three
hours. Since the 20-minute Yogi has neither the time nor the
inclination for meditation, one may ask why he should practise
the Headstand at all. There are several reasons for it.

Before we look at them, a word of warning: From my experience with hundreds of Western students, I have found that
beginners are very keen on the Headstand and that it has almost
an intoxicating effect on them. They are proud of having
learned something which they imagined to be far more difficult.
Their self-confidence increases tremendously. But if a beginner
should decide to stand on his head for ten or even twenty
minutes at the first go, he may well harm himself. I also had
a student who repeated the Headstand a hundred times in one
day. Such exaggerations are positively dangerous. They are
neither in the spirit of Yoga nor in the spirit of this book. The
Headstand should be practised with great care and only after
the preliminary exercises have been mastered and then for not
more than ten to twenty *seconds*. This is quite sufficient for the
first few weeks. Now back to the question of why we practise
the Headstand.

The Headstand is an important aid to evacuation at will and
stimulates the entire circulation It is also a big step towards
deep relaxation.

The effects of the inversion of the body are enormously beneficial. It is self-evident that the replacement of the inner organs

as mentioned on page 59, happens in the inverted position by
itself, especially if the pull of gravity is assisted by deep breathing. The stretched pockets of the colon are emptied and massaged, and in the course of several months the colon gradually
returns to its normal condition. At the same time the enlarged
stomach resumes its normal size which leads to reduced appetite. The effect on the whole digestive system is extremely
strong. Another of the benefits is the reduction of pressure in
the veins of the legs, thereby easing strain on the heart. This
effect can be intensified by circling the feet while in the Headstand, as it acts as a massage of the veins (and the lymphatic
vessels) and helps the flow of the blood back to the heart. For
this reason Indian physicians prescribe the Shoulderstand and
possibly the Headstand for people with heart trouble. Young
people suffering from cold hands and feet find it a real blessing,
since it acts almost immediately.

Another benefit derived from the Headstand is the influence
on the autonomic nervous system. According to the Indian concept, the pituitary gland is favourably affected by an increase
of blood during this posture. The prompt reaction of the blood
vessels is convincing and welcome. Since this effect spreads with
repeated practice to more and more areas of the body, the 20-
minute Yogi has an excellent aid at hand with which he can
direct his circulation to create the desired warmth during deep
relaxation.

THE DANGERS OF THE HEADSTAND

Useful and beneficial as the Headstand can be for most people,
it may possibly spell danger for some. Those who suffer from
severe heart trouble or who had head injuries must under all
circumstances refrain from practising this exercise. The same
holds in the case of sufferers from slipped discs, particularly
if they happen to be in the area of the neck. Hence one should
practise the Dolphin first, as in this posture it is possible to check
up on any hidden defects of the spine. As soon as one feels pain
or hears rasping noises, one must do neither this exercise nor
the Headstand. For those who suffer from disc trouble in the
lumbar region, the Headstand can often be of help and the only

way of inverting the body, for these people are not always able to perform the Shoulderstand. At any rate, in all these cases medical advice *must* be sought. For people with a bad balance and lack of dexterity the Headstand is out of the question. How-. ever, it is recommended for fat people if their blood pressure permits it.

Western students are not infrequently afraid of bursting a blood vessel. It is quite common to experience a rush of blood to the head during the first few attempts, but this soon disappears and should not occur again. Likewise it is quite normal that one should experience the Headstand as refreshing and relaxing. If the rush of blood to the head does not disappear after a while, one should refrain from this exercise. Other reasons for abstaining from practising the Headstand may be scars on the chest or lesions of the diaphragm.

For the majority of exercises the real source of danger lies not in possible contusions etc., but in the non-heeding of the rules. The danger of the Headstand may be compared with the danger of a pedestrian or a motorist. If he crosses the road at the wrong moment or drives on the wrong side of the motorway, he risks his life. But for everybody who observes the traffic rules and uses his common sense, there is no danger whatsoever.

The element of security in performing the Headstand consists in the perfectly symmetrical execution. If one is irresponsible or tense it is inevitable that neck and shoulders are used one-sidedly. The Dolphin serves as a means by which the beginner learns to observe this symmetry. Once he has mastered this aspect, nothing much can happen. He may perhaps once or twice fall against the wall and at worst sprain a shoulder. Or, if he falls down from the Headstand as stiff as a ladder, he might well break a big toe. But even these accidents can be avoided with a little bit of care.

HEADSTAND IN THE SECOND LESSON

In my experience young and athletic middle-aged people are perfectly able to perform the Headstand – against a wall of course – in the second lesson. Others require several lessons before they are ready for it. Most of them are overjoyed when they find they have made progress. The time spent in learning this exercise is never wasted. There is no age limit, although one must be sure of normal blood pressure. My oldest pupil who managed to learn the Headstand was 81 years old. Intending to pay a compliment to an elderly lady who had just learned to stand on her head, I said that this would be a real credit to any grandmother. To my surprise she took objection to my calling her a grandmother, because she was a great-grandmother. It is never too late to begin with Yoga. This woman was not any stiffer than most Western schoolchildren, and hardly anybody improves his flexibility after his school days.

THE DOLPHIN POSTURE AS PREPARATION FOR THE HEADSTAND

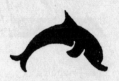

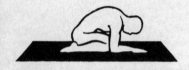

1 Sit in the Thunderbolt posture, bend forward and put the elbows outside the knees with hands flat on the floor.

2 Put the forehead down on the floor and raise the bottom so that the head lies on the crown; do not put the weight on the forehead and do not move the position of the elbows.

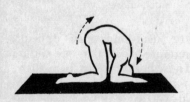

3 Link your hands around the back of the head and spread the little fingers outwards, thus increasing the surface area for the weight distribution. Distribute the weight evenly between elbows and head. Stand on your toes.

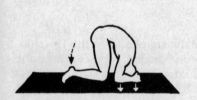

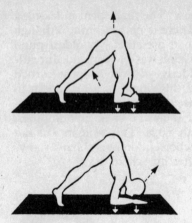

4 Straighten your legs and raise the body with even pressure on the elbows; look between your ankles to secure symmetry. Keep your elbows straight and practise abdominal breathing, with exhalation 'haaa' six times.

5 Bring the pressure entirely on your forearms and slightly raise the head. Once you have mastered this, you can start practising the Headstand.

6 Sink back, kneel and rise up. Before rising, breathe deeply to prevent giddiness.

(To Triangle:)

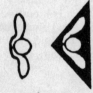

WRONG   RIGHT

Head and elbows form a triangular base supporting the body in the Headstand. The safety of the student relies on the completely even distribution of the weight, which also helps to execute the exercise without much effort.

There are two ways to learn the Headstand; one is difficult, the other easy. The Brahmin literature insists that one should start in the middle of a room and raise both legs simultaneously. The easy way begins with a preparation called the Dolphin, where two-thirds of the weight are carried by the forearms and only one-third rests on the crown of the head.

FROM DOLPHIN TO HEADSTAND

First the student must practise the six phases of the Dolphin. It will be helpful to put a second folded blanket where the triangle of the head and the shoulders rest. This second blanket should not be thicker than six folds. Never practise on a soft cushion or pillow. It is important to practise against a wall or something stable. There should be a few inches space between head and wall.

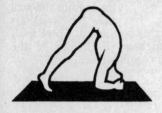

1 Legs are stretched. The weight of the body is distributed evenly on the triangle. For perfect symmetry look between your ankles.

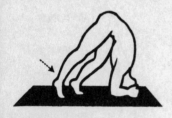

2 The left leg, slightly bent, is placed a little forward while the right leg, which is thrown up afterwards, remains straight. Now the weight is distributed between triangle and bent leg.

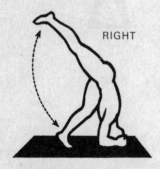

RIGHT

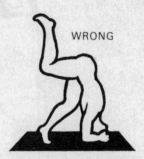

WRONG

3 The right leg is swung straight up and touches the wall.
4 The swinging up is practised several times as a preparation, using alternately the left and the right leg.

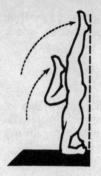

5 The straight leg touches the wall while the other leg is slowly brought up to join it. There must be an even distribution of the weight on the triangle.

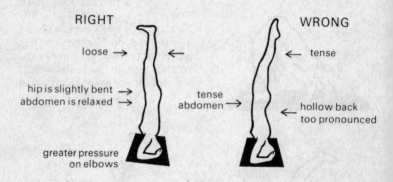

RIGHT   WRONG

loose →   ←   ← tense

hip is slightly bent →   tense   ← hollow back
abdomen is relaxed →   abdomen →   too pronounced

greater pressure
on elbows

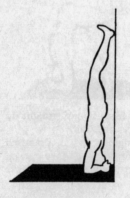

6 Headstand while leaning against a wall. Practise ten to twenty seconds to begin with. On coming down, do not just drop down but bend one knee.

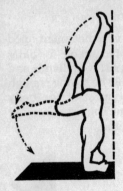

7 Bend the right leg and swing it down. Follow with the left leg.

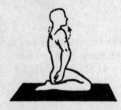

8 Sit in the Thunderbolt posture; raise the right shoulder and drop the left one and vice versa. Continue with rolling the shoulders to counteract possible strain of the shoulder muscles and vertebrae.

Repeat the Headstand two or three times, always following it up with shoulder rolling; at the end relax with the Contemplative Breath.

The usual mistakes of beginners are these: shifting the elbows outwards, thereby putting too much strain on the head; being too far away from the wall with pronounced hollow of the back, or the hands are too near to the wall; they should be about nine inches away from it.

Important: If a student feels giddy after the Headstand he should follow it with deep breathing in the Thunderbolt posture. Only then should he get up. If there is any 'crunching' sound in the neck or in the cervical vertebrae, the exercise must be stopped and the doctor's opinion should be taken. Beginners' muscular pains in the shoulders are usually quite harmless and disappear soon. Do not forget to practise the Contemplative Breath afterwards.

HEADSTAND WITH SUPPORTING HANDS

The second form of the Headstand is usually not mentioned in classical Yoga books. This posture is more suitable for older or overweight people who gain greater support from hands and arms this way. For this exercise the neck must be strong enough not to bend under any circumstances. As most of the body weight presses on the crown of the head one should either use a *hard* cushion or a blanket folded eight times.

Sit in the Thunderbolt posture and bend forward, putting the hands flat on the floor at an even distance from the head. It is important to have an even distribution of the weight on all three points of the triangle – the head and the two hands.

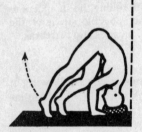

1 As in the Dolphin posture look between your ankles to guarantee perfect symmetry. Then place the left leg slightly forward and bend it.

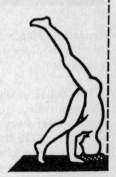

2 Swing the right leg up and leave the left leg on the floor.

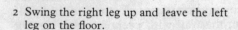

A common mistake with beginners is that they stand too much on the forehead so that the neck is bent back. This is both tiring and dangerous. Another mistake is that the hands are placed too near to the wall, almost at both sides of the head, and therefore the triangle is too flat to support the bodily weight evenly.

Important: This variation should not be practised by children or youths under the age of 16.

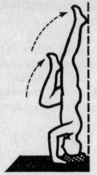

3 When the right leg touches the wall draw the left leg up as well. A slightly hollow back is permitted. Ensure that there is an even distribution of the weight on all three points of the triangle.

4 In the free Headstand the weight is slightly more on the front part of the crown of the head.

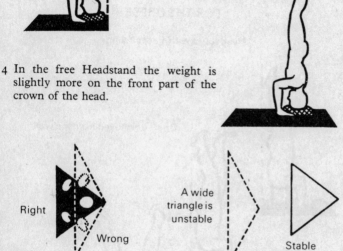

Right

Wrong

A wide triangle is unstable

Stable

HEADSTAND FOR OVERWEIGHT PEOPLE

The Headstand with hand support is easy for short sturdy people with strong shoulders and short arms. Corpulent men should not shy away from this exercise provided that their blood pressure allows it. The Headstand is more athletic than any other posture and is best suited to their need to express physical strength. As overweight people usually suffer from constipation and mostly have stiff ankles and circulatory disturbances in the legs, the Headstand with foot circling is the strongest means of correction.

Though the Headstand is more athletic than other Yoga postures it does not mean that it is strenuous. One should be capable of retaining this posture without any trembling for several minutes and be able to speak normally whilst in it. However, the beginner should not speak while doing the Headstand.

FOR THE OBESE

Headstand with Foot circling

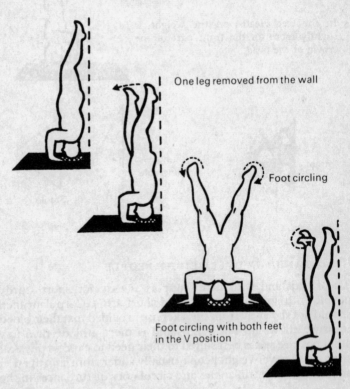

One leg removed from the wall

Foot circling

Foot circling with both feet in the V position

FREE HEADSTAND

Before starting the more difficult version of the free Headstand, it should have been practised for several months against a wall or wardrobe. After all, the essence of Yoga exercises is not acrobatics but the effect on the nerve centres, the inner organs and the circulatory system.

If the student wants to practise the Headstand without any support in the middle of the room there is one technique which will help him considerably. By inserting the little fingers under the crown of the head in such a way that they increase the supporting area of the triangle, they prevent the neck from bending backwards, which frightens many beginners.

Free Headstand

From the Dolphin posture

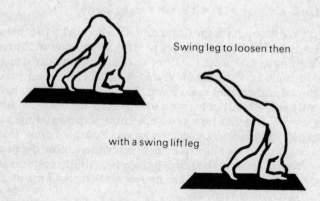

Swing leg to loosen then

with a swing lift leg

FROM THE DOLPHIN POSTURE

The weight is taken off the right leg which is then swung upwards. The other leg is brought up slowly. It is a relief to cross the feet when remaining in the Headstand for a longer period.

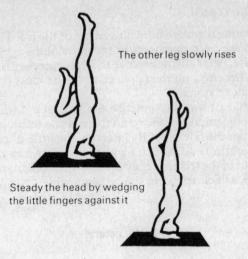

The other leg slowly rises

Steady the head by wedging
the little fingers against it

LOOK AT YOURSELF FROM A DISTANCE

Prepare yourself for the Contemplative Breath by practising the
Headstand twice and then try to imagine yourself in the following situation: You are the director of a big company which you
have built up over many years of hard work. You have developed and created everything. Just assume that you have recently retired and only come to the office for your enjoyment,
as it were. Imagine how you walk through the buildings, greet-
ing old friends, clerks and workmen. You are happy that you
do not need to give any more orders for this is now the business
of your successor. The burden of responsibility rests no longer
on your shoulders. You are merely a visitor looking at all the
many activities from afar.

Become detached from your feelings and wishes. Permit your
body to carry on its own business. Permit your eyes to rest in
the way they want and your blood vessels and organs to relax
and dilate. Let your body bask in the sensation of relaxation.
Act like a painter who every so often steps back from the canvas
to look at his work from a distance; only then can he detect
if something is wrong.

Practise the Contemplative Breath. Follow the cold and warm flow of your breath and feel how shoulders and back gain in weight. Feel the warmth behind your eyes – in your hands and arms and in the solar plexus. Observe your body as if it was somebody else's. Feel and enjoy the wonderfully relaxing and refreshing warmth.

UDDHIYANA-BANDHA (*Uddhiyana-bandha* – 'upwards lock') OR THE ABDOMINAL LIFT

A further exercise in the programme of the 20-minute Yogi which is very beneficial is the so-called Abdominal Lift. During exhalation, as a result of the suction created by pulling up the abdomen, the whole intestines and inner organs are raised. This effects an overall stretching and massaging. The heart is compressed, and this might cause a short attack of giddiness which is quite harmless and soon passes. However, it is necessary to observe one's reaction to this exercise and to follow the instructions conscientiously.

The Abdominal Lift is performed after two or three repetitions of the Headstand, since during the Headstand the intestines have already been shifted and prepared for the suction. The result in the Headstand is due to the gravitational pull, whilst in the Abdominal Lift it is achieved through energetic exhalation and the contraction and lift of the diaphragm.

Important: This exercise is prohibited for pregnant women. You should also never practise it with a full stomach nor repeat it more than two or three times. In between each lift one should taken ten slow breaths.

This exercise is one of the most successful means of counteracting constipation. Although overweight people will hardly notice the contraction of the abdomen, this should be no reason to neglect it.

The following exercise serves as a preparation for the abdominal lift:

Strictly speaking, the Abdominal Lift is nothing else but an energetic 'haaa' exhalation which usually is performed while standing. The Shoulderstand serves as a preparation for it. This

SLIM   OBESE

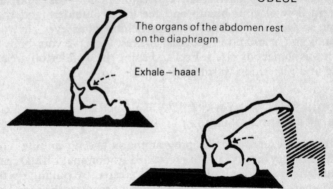

The organs of the abdomen rest
on the diaphragm

Exhale – haaa!

exercise consists of four phases. People with operational scars
on the abdomen or lesions of the diaphragm are allowed to perform this exercise only with the permission of their doctor.

Phase I: Stand with legs apart and loose knees. Raise both arms and
             inhale through the mouth.
             Fill the lungs as if you were diving. You need a supply of
             oxygen as during the next two phases no breath is taken
             in.

Phase II: Exhale strongly through the open mouth. Bend forward,
             put your hands above the knees and press the trunk to the
             thighs.
             Squeeze the air from the lungs as if you were trying to keep
             no air in at all; the head is almost between the knees.

Phase III: Do not inhale. Stretch the body by straightening arms and
             legs, but keep the back round and the pelvis forward as if
             you were pulling in your tail.
             Suck in the abdomen (do not press). The nearly empty
             lungs act like a suction pump and draw the contents of the
             abdomen upwards. Wait for a few seconds while pressing
             the chin against the chest.

Phase IV: Inhale gradually by sucking the air through pursed lips as
             if you wanted to whistle inside with the intake of the air.
             Do not open the throat so that the air can rush into the
             body (this is dangerous). Slowly allow the abdomen to sink
             and inflate like a balloon (this is important for the peris-
             talsis). Straighten up and exhale. Sit down. Take ten
             breaths.

The Abdominal Lift

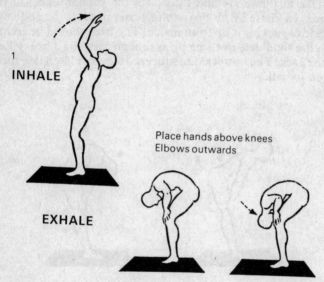

1

INHALE

EXHALE

Place hands above knees
Elbows outwards

2. Open mouth and continue exhalation

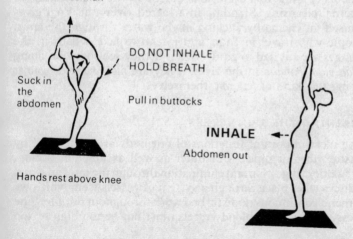

3. The Coalman

Suck in
the
abdomen

Hands rest above knee

DO NOT INHALE
HOLD BREATH

Pull in buttocks

INHALE

Abdomen out

Common mistakes of the beginner: he is inclined to inhale by mistake in Phase III and thus loses the suction effect of the thorax. In Phase IV he also wrongly tries to press the abdomen instead of sucking it up from inside. The back should be arched with the shoulders pressing up as though carrying a heavy load on the back. The buttocks are squeezed together like a dog tucking in its tail.

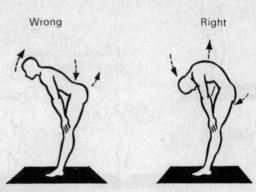

Wrong   Right

In India the Abdominal Lift is considered the most important Hatha-Yoga exercise for the beginner. In the Brahmin schools of India this exercise is taught as one of the means of internal cleansing. Standing in a sacred river, the Yogi gives himself an enema by sucking in the water through the anus. People who travel in India and intend to take a bath in the Ganges are advised to go upstream if they see someone doing *uddhiyana-bandha* in the river. They are also warned against trying this kind of 'enema' themselves.

TRAINING THE SPHINCTERS

The most important functions of our body are performed by elastic tubes or pipes. The outer as well as inner breathing, circulation, digestion and elimination through the intestines and kidneys takes place through a system of vessels from which we demand continuous undisturbed work throughout our life. The pressure inside the blood vessels must not be too high or too low, and the lungs and intestines must not be distended. All valves must remain efficient often for more than 80 years. When in elderly people the elasticity of the vessels begins to give, one must ask oneself if this could not have been prevented or could still be improved. After all, we expect much more service from them than from any car tyre.

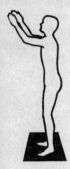

1 Stand relaxed with heels together, toes pointing outwards. Raise your arms with open hands and inhale simultaneously through the nose. Hold the breath for a moment.

2 Exhale forcibly through the mouth and at the same time bring the arms down, clench your fists and practise the chinlock. Contract the buttocks, pull in the rectum and contract the bladder. This is easier if simultaneously one contracts arm and leg muscles and presses the heels together as well as bending the shoulders forward. Remain for a moment in this contraction.

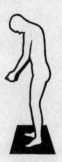

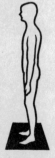

3 Relax, straighten up and inhale through the nose.
Note: If you are told that the bladder cannot be contracted, try it nevertheless. You will see that it works although it may take some time.

Besides incontinence which sometimes troubles elderly people, the opposite can be equally disturbing: an enlarged prostrate in men can prevent the elimination of urine. In India a special exercise is taught as an effective prevention for this. The training of the sphincters in the rectum which is part of that exercise is also very effective in cases of haemorrhoids and prolapse of the anus. It is of course best to take this up in one's daily programme while still in the fifties. This exercise for both the bladder and the sphincter of the rectum, is performed whilst standing and consists of three phases: inhalation, contraction with exhalation, relaxation with inhalation.

X

Yoga for the Over-Sixties

GROWING OLD OR AGEING

There is an enormous difference between growing old and ageing. Growing old is inevitable, even for a Yogi. Ageing, however, has its own laws and depends partly on physical and partly on mental factors. This can only be understood when one takes into account the constitution, environmental influences and the intelligence as well as the character of the individual. The purely physiological processes consist mainly in the displacement and the wear and tear of organs, the condition of the spine and the auto-intoxication. One person may age prematurely, while another seems to stay young for ever. In other words – ageing is a relative concept. The process of growing older can be speeded up or slowed down, and there is even a possibility of a certain rejuvenation.

THE POSSIBILITY OF RELATIVE REJUVENATION

For a great number of people who are still in their best years, the possibility of rejuvenation, even if only relatively, is of great importance. In order to understand what this means, one must realise what vitality implies. Vitality is dependent on several factors. It needs a healthy constitution, certain character traits such as courage and patience and such acquired abilities as judgement and education.

A healthy constitution, such as a countryman might possess, does not necessarily imply that he has great vitality. Let us assume that a countryman with his friend from the city is involved in an accident. The latter has a far weaker physical constitution. Both lose a leg. The one with the greater vitality will be able to adjust himself more easily to this new situation and quickly gets used to an artificial leg. While he is able to continue his work and so pull his weight, the other will walk on crutches, possibly for the rest of his life, simply because he is lacking some mental component of his vitality. And this might well be the countryman who otherwise is as strong as an ox. As any physician will confirm, vitality is a decisive factor in the healing of broken bones and the overcoming of post-operative shock. Vitality represents the total picture of the state of health of a person and is the most significant criterion in rejuvenation.

THE THREE CURVES OF VITALITY

Let us take the example of a man in his 40s whose vitality curve has dropped to a position corresponding with that of a 55-year-old. In other words, he has aged a full 15 years before his time. This is not at all rare. Now if he should manage to get his vitality curve to rise again to the level of a 40-year-old, he would have rejuvenated himself by those 15 years. This oscillation can be seen in curve A of the following diagram.

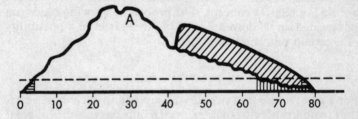

Theoretical considerations demand that the vitality curve rises between the time of birth and the twenty-fifth year in an unbroken line. There it should remain for about ten years horizontally and after that begin to decline, ending approximately with the eightieth birthday. However, in reality the curve looks quite different. Every illness delays the ascent and causes a notch in the curve. On the horizontal line illness shows up as a dent. Infections and accidents from which an ageing person does not fully recover accelerate the decline of his health, which is shown in the curve in the form of steps. The broken line indicates the likely continuation of the curve without the rejuvenation process. The shaded area stands for the gain in efficiency and as a result of rejuvenation.

THE IDEAL VITALITY CURVE

It is possible to map the vitality of a physically and mentally healthy and disciplined person. His curve will have neither dents nor steps. Since he remains always on the highest possible level of vitality there can be no question of a rejuvenation for him. The perfect man could easily live to an age of 120 years or more. The idea of surviving all our grandchildren may not be attractive, but the graphic depiction of the ideal case is more than an academic game. This will become evident when we super-impose and compare curve A of the normal contemporary, curve B of the ideal man and curve C of a person on a low physical and mental level.

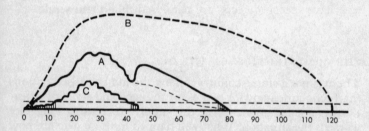

Curve C is by no means a far-fetched speculation. Its contorted appearance with numerous kinks rising to little height and soon declining, corresponds with the low vitality of the sick and undernourished. People who belong to this group often are plagued by vermin and may suffer from one infection after another, unable to recuperate from any of their many illnesses. They presumably compose one-third of mankind. Their vitality curve is a horrible reality.

THE MIDDLE PATH

Somewhere between the minimal curve C and the optimal curve B we can trace our individual curve A. Sometime between 60 and 70 we cross the threshold to enter a new phase of life. The possibility of rejuvenation becomes increasingly reduced. In this case one may ask whether there is any purpose to continue with exercises at all. If there is no longer any chance of rejuvenation, how can we possibly increase our vitality? The over-60s compose about 15–20 per cent of modern industrialised countries. A considerable number live below yet another threshold in various stages of dependency and helplessness. Their increasing demands exhaust the means and possibilities of private and public institutions concerned with the care of the old. Against their will they have regressed and become like children who must be dressed, fed and protected. When an old person happens to forsake his independence, he also loses an essential element of his personality. His own recollections, goals and preferences are lost. Even lower lie those tragic cases of old people who have speech defects, are paralysed, blind and senile.

THE CONTRIBUTION OF THE OLD

There is not a single country among the industrialised nations in which the demand for homes for the aged and similar institutions is not far greater than the supply. Increasing longevity worsens the situation. What will happen to those who are now in their 40s or 50s is easily predictable. 'Yoga over 60' is more than an attempt to adjust to the inevitable. It is the honourable intention of people to live above the line of independence so that they may continue to enjoy life and at the same time not become a burden to their family and the state.

Elderly people are often put off by the thought that there is an age limit to Yoga. If there is such a limit at all, it is more likely to exist on the level of the 12-year-old. It is not recommended to introduce boys of that age-group to Yoga. They are too hasty, their spines are too weak and they do not take it seriously enough. There is no prohibition for older people, and the only thing they might regret later on is the fact that they did not take up Yoga sooner.

'Yoga over 60' aims at the preservation of one's personality and independence. This is mainly a question of the sustenance of the vital functions, the most important of which is thinking. Then follow breathing, digestion, circulation and sleep. To the immediate target belongs also the persistent effort to keep limbs and spine flexible. The daily relaxation is meant to lead to physical and mental experiences which bring enjoyment into the life of the elderly, and perhaps even further development.

However, all vital functions are directed by the autonomic nervous system over which we have no direct control. Although we are able to bend and stretch a finger at will, the sphincter which closes or opens the rectum is beyond our control.

The aim of this book is to make the reader realise that with the help of breathing exercises and a daily programme of postures and relaxation he can learn to influence the autonomous nervous system indirectly and thus improve his control over digestion, the activity of the heart and glands as well as his sleep. It is not possible to bully the autonomous nervous system, but one can learn to entice it in a round-about way and invite it to function properly.

Yoga for the over-60s consists of the same three disciplines – breathing, posture, relaxation – though in a more selective way. The Yogi over 60 who has done his daily exercises for a number of years knows from experience that he cannot do everything a much younger person is able to cope with. He finds that after an accident his spine is much less flexible than before or that his knees are stiffer. Some old scars begin to hurt in certain postures, not to mention occasional twinges of arthritis or sciatica, should he suffer from either.

Yet there should be no difficulty to find exercises suitable for yourself. The Yogi over 60 should not grieve about his limited possibilities but should enjoy the fact that he can substitute a valuable contribution by precision and concentration on the finer details.

MAN, THE LATE DEVELOPER

Man takes longer than any other creature to reach full maturity. A diploma is no guarantee of maturity. A driving licence does not make a person a responsible motorist, and no amount of academic training produces an experienced physician or lawyer. A really mature man under 30 is a rarity. The great advantage of the Yogi over 60 is his spiritual maturity. His mind is (or should be) such that it seeks to integrate opposites and fill gaps, and therefore gives him the opportunity and possibility of crystallising his personality and of experiencing fulfilment and joy.

Education makes a person not only more sensitive and inwardly richer, it also opens for the mature man completely new dimensions of thought and enjoyment. The Yogi over 60 has left behind the pursuits of youth and now has the unique opportunity of entering the sphere of the deeper spiritual experiences during his deep relaxation. Thus the door to meditation opens for him. Older people are often better prepared and equipped for meditation than the younger generation. It is quite possible that their spiritual development receives a new impetus which takes them far beyond the field of Hatha-Yoga. If this happens, then 'Yoga over 60' has truly found its culmination.

THE DAILY PROGRAMME

Whereas the Oriental tends to frown upon any fixed method, most Western readers are only able to utilise a large amount of information when it is put together systematically. Hence I feel that it is justifiable to put what has been said so far into clear schedules which are intended as suggestions. Nobody need do all the exercises listed or even stick to the times given for them. A closer examination of the various series of exercises will show that there are a number of pauses inserted which must not be omitted. If one cannot do the Shoulderstand twice, one does it once. Furthermore, nobody should worry if he cannot do one or another exercise perfectly or not at all.

The efficiency of Yoga does not lie in the perfection of an exercise nor in one's failure to acquire perfect flexibility, but in the quiet, patient and purposeful practice. If one's body is too stiff in the morning, there is no reason why one should not do the exercises in the late afternoon. One should always practise with leisure, in a positive frame of mind and by keeping sufficiently long pauses. It also is part of the rejuvenation programme to weigh oneself once a week. Those who neglect to do this, may end up with a bad conscience which only impedes progress. To get rid of the first few pounds is most difficult of all, but with practice one will be rewarded with a definite rejuvenation demonstrated by a loss of weight. Another way of rejuvenation is through deep relaxation.

XI

Twenty-Minute Yoga Programme

SEQUENCE OF EXERCISES FOR SLIM PEOPLE

Exercise Name and Description	Number of times	Mental Focus	Duration (seconds)
BREATHING			
(a) Complete Breathing in Thunderbolt posture	6	Peace and strength	60–90
(b) *Bhastrika* in Thunderbolt posture	6 left 6 right	Cleansing	60
LOOSENING UP			
(a) Windmill	6 forward 6 backward	Loosening of shoulders	60
(b) Swinging Through	6	Swinging	30
(c) Triangular posture	3 both sides	Stretching	30
ASANAS In prone position:			
(a) Contemplative Breath with knees up	1	Space between eyebrows	15
(b) Half Shoulderstand, 6 times soundless 'haaa' breath and rolling down, Contemplative Breath	2	Abdomen	90
(c) Half Shoulderstand with Foot Circling, Plough, rolling down, Contemplative Breath	1	Solar plexus	90

Exercise Name and Description	Number of times	Mental Focus	Duration (seconds)
In abdominal position:			
(d) Cobra	3	Kidneys	30
Pause	1	Small of back	10
(e) Locust	3	Back	30
Pause	1	Small of back	10
(f) Bow	2	Kidneys	30
Pause	1	Small of back	10
On the head:			
(g) Contemplative Breath	1	Peace	15
(h) Headstand from Dolphin ca. 15 secs each, rolling shoulders	2	Abdomen	60
(i) Contemplative Breath	1	Abdomen	30
Standing:			
(k) Abdominal Lift, 10 secs each time with pause (sitting)	2	Abdomen	60
(l) Contemplative Breath	1	Warmth	60

SEQUENCE OF EXERCISES FOR UNCOORDINATED AND WEAK PEOPLE

People of this group and those with heart diseases should first consult their doctor before taking up this programme.

Exercise Name and Description	Number of times	Mental Focus	Duration (seconds)
BREATHING			
(a) Complete Breathing sitting on a stool	6	Peace	30–60
(b) *Bhastrika*, sitting	3 left 3 right	Cleansing of sinuses	60
LOOSENING UP			
(a) Windmill	6 forward 6 backward	Loosening of shoulders	30
(b) Triangular Posture	3	Stretching	30

Exercise Name and Description	Number of times	Mental Focus	Duration (seconds)
ASANAS			
In prone position:			
(a) Contemplative Breath with knees up	1	Concentration on space between eyebrows	120
(b) Drawing up of leg	3 each		
(c) Contemplative Breath	1	Abdomen	120
(d) Foot Circling	2	Ankles, calves	10–20
(e) Contemplative Breath	1	Legs	120
In abdominal position:			
(f) Cobra	2–3	Abdomen	20
Pause with shallow breath	1		20
(g) Locust, raise one leg only	3 each	Back	30
Pause		Kidneys	20
(h) Foot Circling	2	Ankles	20
In prone position:			
(i) Contemplative Breath	1	Warmth	120

For bedridden people:
Contemplative Breath in prone position with drawn-up knees and deep abdominal breathing

mornings before breakfast	1	10 mins
midday before meal	1	10 mins
evenings before going to sleep	1	10 mins
at night (for insomnia and depression)	repeat for a longer time	

SEQUENCE OF EXERCISES FOR OBESE PEOPLE

Exercise Name and Description	Number of times	Mental Focus	Duration (seconds)
BREATHING			
(a) Complete Breathing kneeling post	6	Peace and strength	60
(b) *Bhastrika*, sitting	6 left 6 right	Cleansing of sinuses	60

Exercise Name and Description	Number of times	Mental Focus	Duration (seconds)
LOOSENING UP			
(a) Windmill	6 forward 6 backward	Loosening of shoulders	60
(b) Swinging Through	6	Swinging	30
(c) Triangular Posture, with legs apart	3	Stretching	30
ASANAS			
In prone position:			
(a) Contemplative Breath with knees up	1	Space between eyebrows	20
(b) Half Shoulderstand, feet on back of chair, soundless 'haaa' breath, rolling down, Contemplative Breath	2	Abdomen	90
(c) Half Shoulderstand, with Foot Circling, rolling down, Contemplative Breath	2	Solar plexus	90
(d) Bending Forward, trying to touch the toes, Contemplative Breath	2	Abdomen	60
In abdominal position (with pillow):			
(e) Cobra Pause	3 1	Kidneys	40
(f) Locust Pause	3	Small of back	40
(g) Contemplative Breath	1	Peace, space between eyebrows	30
(h) Dolphin, with 'haaa' exhalation	1	Abdomen	20
(i) Contemplative Breath	1	Abdomen	30
(k) Headstand with palms flat on the floor, 'haaa' exhalation during posture	1 or 2	Abdomen	30
(l) Contemplative Breath	1	Warmth	60

XII

Self-Help Through Relaxation

RELAXATION – AN EXPERIENCE

It is a good idea to go to a sauna and afterwards have a massage. However, you should not try to lose more than one pound at a time. Excellent as sauna and massage are, they are not really acts of self-help. The wellbeing after a bath or massage is bought, not worked for, and will therefore not last for long. It is surprising how few people are able to see the difference between being actively or merely passively interested in their health. These people are quite convinced that they do something for themselves when they go to the sauna or a masseur. But all that happens is that something is being done to them.

ON NOT-DOING AND NON-DOING

For the busy man in the West it is a long way from doing to non-doing. His whole life is orientated towards action and he looks down on all passive attitudes. He regards inactivity as sinful. Yet one should not overlook that the active Western approach is complemented by the Eastern approach of passivity or non-doing which is not the same as doing nothing. The latter is by no means unproductive. Non-doing is not the same as indolence. It is a conscious decision to avoid aggressive activity, and as such it is a form of mental self-discipline and hence a kind of work. The insight into the value of non-doing is decisive for a proper comprehension of the Eastern wisdom and also of the deep relaxation of Yoga.

The validity of a conscious passivity is best demonstrated in Oriental games such as chess or in teachings such as the Japanese Judo (also called Jiu-Jitsu), Karate or Zen archery, etc. They emphasise the possibility of victory over the opponent by yielding and being passive and thus using one's own strength to bring him down. Eastern politics has a predilection for the art of non-doing and passive resistance.

It is important to understand this difference really well if one wants to get on with the relaxation of Yoga. Relaxation is a kind of mental discipline which requires simultaneous activity and passivity. Those who understand this hold the key to relaxation and the beginnings of meditation.

BODILY ACTIVITY DURING MENTAL PASSIVITY

The Orientals are quite familiar with these things. They are not surprised when they see somebody in a trance state or under hypnosis. The hypnotised subject receives orders passively and then executes them actively with his body. About forty years ago it was popular at shows to give demonstrations of the powers of hypnosis. People were asked to come up on the platform where they were hypnotised. Then they were ordered, for example, to play the cello. To the general merriment the person then began to play devotedly – with umbrella and broom stick.

Although such performances are rare today, the number of 'hypnotised' subjects has increased. However, the form of hypnosis has changed: It has turned into a chronic disease of ruthless self-exploitation. Hundreds of thousands of victims of self-hypnosis can be found in factories and firms and in almost every family. These are the people who never relax. They rush along as if they were driven. They do not allow themselves to have a holiday and even fill their spare time with hectic activities. This kind of self-hypnosis is partly due to the false mental attitude that every activity must be an order given by oneself, which leads to the common phenomenon of forcing things. This is nothing but cruelty to oneself. In contrast with this is the Oriental attitude which can best be described as introspective.

DE-HYPNOTISATION THROUGH INTROSPECTION

Introspection is an experience during deep relaxation. It is the exact opposite of yelling orders at oneself. It consists of an inward listening that demands a high degree of attention for which most people are unprepared. There are two types of concentration. Typical of the West is the concentration of efficiency. We acquire it at school and intensify it during our working life. The concentration of the Easterner, on the other hand, is more of a contemplation. Its fulfilment lies in subjective experiences and the termination of self-hypnosis and not in external results which can be measured and expressed in figures or charts.

We are largely blind to this way of looking at life, and this is the source of many undesirable consequences. We have become unable to understand the signals of our own body and try our best to ignore and suppress its protests, if necessary by way of chemicals. We take pills for headaches, sleeplessness, heart trouble and indigestion. The relief is only temporary and the drugging has to be repeated possibly with increasingly stronger dosages. Then there comes a point when the body collapses and refuses to cooperate in this cold war against itself. Often this breakdown is the beginning of an interest in relaxation.

RESTING POSE

How are we to relax? The first step is to lie down as comfortably as possible. Strangely enough, few people manage to do this. Most of the students require exact instructions before they are able to lie down relaxed for a period of twenty to forty minutes without getting a backache. Yoga books usually ask the student to stretch himself flat out on a blanket in the manner depicted in the first drawing. This is only possible for those who have neither a round nor a hollow back. A round back, especially in obese people, causes the head to sink back in the typical snoring position. This only emphasises the hollow of the back in the lumbar region. Hence this position is uncomfortable for most Western students.

The neck should not lie on the cushion; the shoulder-blades should rest on the blanket and the back should be flat. Placing the hands on the thighs makes the experience of warmth easier.

UNCOMFORTABLE

I. Exaggerated

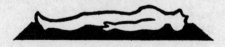

II. Unsuitable for the obese; invites snoring

Hollow back   Round back

COMFORTABLE

III. For the slim

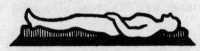

Mattress

IV. For the obese

The heavier you are – the thicker the mattress and cushion

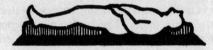

Mattress

Now the back lies flat

Being kind to oneself includes covering the body with a blanket during relaxation. Needless to say one should practise in a temperate room and if possible on a carpet. To cover the body helps to achieve the initially rather weak stirrings of the warmth. Furthermore, it is best to practise in a darkened room or to lie down in such a way that the eyes are not exposed to strong light.

PRELUDE TO DEEP RELAXATION

Deep relaxation is not something that one can *do*. It is an experience composed of several acts and a series of shorter scenes, rather like a play. Nature is the author of the play and the body is the stage. Our mind is the audience. But the simile is not perfect: For whereas the audience in a theatre is stationary, the mind should wander throughout the body and remain conscious of all the bodily sensations. The exertion connected with this is purely mental. Therefore relaxation can be called a mental discipline. The student should first direct his attention to the breath, since, as has been said already, it is easier to concentrate on a flowing movement than on a static point. The first act of the play of relaxation is entitled 'experience of heaviness'.

EXERCISE: DEEP RELAXATION (Duration about 15–20 minutes)

Close your eyes. Start with the Contemplative Breath. The tongue should be relaxed. The knees are not drawn up as usually in the Contemplative Breath but the legs lie flat on the mat or blanket. If a mattress is used it should reach up to the buttocks. The heels should touch and the toes point outwards. After a few minutes of breathing we observe how a heaviness flows into hands and feet as if it came from outside the body. This sensation of weight is not commanded but comes by itself. It slowly spreads over the entire body. The back sinks deeper and flatter onto the floor till one gets the impression that it has become flat as a pan or bowl. This particular sensation plays an important role in the third stage of relaxation.

By placing the legs on the mattress the pelvis is tilted

upwards, which invites the inner organs to fall back into their proper position. We direct our mind to the abdomen and observe whatever processes occur there. We invite our arms and legs to become like dough or like a sack of sand or to become fluid. This will create the sensation that the muscles have become heavier and melting. They become as heavy as logs. We begin to think that we shall be unable to get up ever again.

Then we come back very slowly. We allow our legs and arms to lose the sensation of heaviness. We may have the impression that our limbs are fused with our body to a single whole. We invite them to regain their independence. We tell them that they can move again. Then, after a few deep breaths, we open our eyes. Relaxation is completed. We note down the duration of the exercise.

Warning: It is wrong and dangerous to pull out of deep relaxation too suddenly. For this reason, before starting take the receiver off the telephone or settle any expected phone calls rather than be interrupted, as this can be a shock to the nervous system.

WHEN TO RELAX?

Many books on Yoga agree that relaxation is best practised after the morning exercises, but this is a time when most people can hardly spare a minute. Also one should not relax with a full stomach. This prevents some people from trying relaxation altogether, which of course is quite wrong. If one cannot produce ideal conditions, one has to be satisfied with the second best and perhaps relax after lunch. In my experience this is the only time many housewives have for a little leisure. Artists, like singers, actors or musicians, may find another time more suitable.

RELAXATION OR A NAP?

Few people are lucky enough to be able to afford a nap after lunch. For working people this may be possible perhaps only once a week or month on a Saturday or Sunday. Then they mostly sleep from sheer exhaustion and wake up with a need for some stimulant like coffee or tea. The remaining sluggishness is an almost painful experience. From the point of view of the Hatha-Yogi such cat naps are out of date; they belong to the many Western malpractices.

A beginner might need about 30 minutes to relax properly, and an advanced student could achieve the same results in half that time. However, when both open their eyes, they have a feeling of being greatly refreshed. The lunchtime snooze is merely a sip at the source of recreation which makes the body hunger for more. During sleep body and mind are passive while in relaxation the body is passive but the mind is active. It is just this mental activity which speeds up the circulation and the various metabolic processes on which relaxation is based. A personal experiment will easily show that one gets up from relaxation fresh and wide awake.

Many people who are continually exhausted find that they fall asleep during relaxation. This happens mostly when the sensation of warmth occurs. Falling asleep during relaxation is both wrong and annoying. Wrong, because it leads not to recreation but sluggishness, and annoying because it can happen that one forgets to wake up in time. Luckily there are certain measures one can take to prevent it. The first thing one can do is to place a clock in sight from which one can read the time without having to turn the head, but simply by opening the eyes. This will not interrupt the process of relaxation. Moreover, one should follow the breathing rhythm. As long as one inhales slowly and deeply one will stay awake, but if the breath gets shorter it indicates that mental concentration wanes and that, before long, one is going to fall asleep. One should get used to listening to the slow, audible rhythm of the breath.

The more advanced student sometimes experiences the reverse, namely that from sleep he glides into a deeper state of relaxation, but such experiences are likely to happen only as a result of fasting or moderate eating habits.

FORMING HABITS

Relaxation of about 20 minutes should become a daily habit. This will guarantee success in the form of an increase in energy and freshness. Finally one is able to experience heaviness and warmth with the same automatic certainty with which the skilled motorist switches gears.

The more regularly you practise, the quicker and surer you can expect to make progress. We have all the help from our body which is only too keen to enjoy the comfort and peace of relaxation. It is not the body which must learn to relax but our undisciplined mind, and it is the mind which has failed us when we fall asleep during relaxation or are altogether unable to relax. Therefore we must give the mind sufficient time to get into this new experience; we should not discontinue the relaxation too early and afterwards complain that it does not work. Only the master experiences the deepest stages within a few minutes, but mastership requires long, regular daily practice. If we interrupt this regularity, it is inevitable that we suffer a setback.

INNER RESISTANCES

It would be quite unrealistic to ignore the resistances which some students are up against. There are many hurdles to overcome, foremost the neurotic urge to control. The inner resistances which do not proceed from the body but from the mind, prevent exactly those people from relaxing who most urgently need relaxation. Some people are simply afraid that it is nothing but an Eastern mumbo-jumbo. They may have read exciting books about secret India and now fear to become bewitched or hypnotised or to behave badly while in relaxation.

These poor people can be helped when they understand that relaxation is after all a gift of nature and not an invention of the Yogis. Yoga only shows how to use what nature has given to us while we were still in the cradle. There is no cause for a bad conscience except when one fails to practise regularly. Relaxation is more than a short-term blessing or enjoyment. It purifies and detoxicates the body. It should be part of one's daily habits like brushing one's teeth or washing. Not to relax is a great sin against yourself. A vivid example are all those people who age prematurely and are continually exhausted and morose; they have no joy in life or in their work and stagger towards an early grave. Hence – relax and live longer.

EXERCISE: THE EXPERIENCE OF HEAVINESS IN TRUNK AND HEAD

Lie down, close your eyes and begin to breathe slowly and rhythmically with the abdomen. Imagine that with each inhalation a cold stream reaches the area behind your eyes while a warm stream flows out with the exhalation. Now as before observe how your limbs get heavier and the body seems to melt. Then bring your awareness back to breathing. Observe the rhythmic flow of the breath from cold to warm and vice versa.

There is a particular place behind the eyes in the middle of the head which becomes distinctly warmer. A pleasant sensation spreads around the eyes and inside the nose. This sensation is both calming and purifying. The eyes feel as if they were falling back into their sockets. They feel as if they grew bigger and heavier – like glass marbles glowing from within. This must not be a strain on the physical eyes but introspection carried out with the mental eyes. Once we have grown accustomed to this kind of introspection we can also understand the expression of the Indian, Chinese and Japanese sculptures depicting holy men in meditation. Then we will realise that Yoga meditation cannot be learned without having first been introduced to the art of introspection. This exercise should be done for about 20 minutes.

DEEP RELAXATION FOR INSOMNIA

It is quite possible that the Indian teaching of locking out all unwanted thoughts contains important hints for all those people who suffer from insomnia. There are as many methods to overcome sleeplessness as there are causes for it. Among older people and those confined to bed who suffer from it, one reason is very often a lack of activity. While their mind longs for rest, their body is not tired enough and wants to be active, perhaps only to relieve a disturbance of circulation. In such cases a quarter of an hour of deep abdominal breathing will often bring about the necessary degree of tiredness and thus the much desired sleep.

Another frequent cause of insomnia is the heavy demand made on the digestive system through overeating. According to Indian texts this causes pressure on the solar plexus. While we in the West seek relief mainly through bought remedies, the Eastern people rely on abdominal breathing. Hence the advice of Yoga experts to decrease the pressure on the solar plexus by at least 15 minutes of energetic abdominal breathing. The strong massage of the abdomen lessens and shifts the pressure. As breathing relieves the pressure, sleep becomes possible.

Breathing in relaxation has yet another beneficial effect, namely the detoxication of the body. Easterners are convinced that not only exhaustion but also excitement leads to an accumulation of toxic substances in the body. Indeed the tiredness of the exhausted has much in common with the symptoms of poisoning. The Japanese think that rage, for instance, is caused by a toxic substance in the body which they call 'rage substance'. They believe that it is responsible for a person's outburst of anger and that it can only be eliminated by breathing. Too much of this 'rage substance' can decide the result of a fight in a duel with sword or bow, and it is a very ancient tactic in the East to insult one's opponent before the fight in order to make him lose his self-control. For if he gets excited his hand will shake.

The Indian view goes even beyond that. They maintain that every emotional excitement such as fear, jealousy or shame produces an accumulation of toxic matter in the body which has the purpose of deepening the breath and of preparing the body for the fight. Western medical opinion will probably agree that Adrenalin, produced by the Adrenal glands (the Adrenal glands are attached to the top of both kidneys), is a crisis hormone. It is ejected into the blood stream at moments of danger and causes a constriction of the vessels and an immediate alarm situation in the whole body. Hence the pale look of a shocked person and his short, jerky breathing. A fair dosage of this crisis hormone will also prevent sleep, as do coffee and other stimulants.

BREATHING AWAY THE DISTURBANCE

Whether there is only one or many toxic substances in the body, they are all eliminated through deep breathing, particularly when done in deep relaxation. Whether this happens by way of oxidation or by any other process remains to be decided. Especially effective in relaxation is the Four-Bar Breath. It is a strange experience to observe how anger or any other negative emotion flows out of the body. On the other hand, one can now understand why people with shallow breathing are overcharged with toxic matter and therefore usually are bad sleepers. This detoxication belongs to the most profound experiences of Hatha-Yoga. It cannot really be put into words but must be experienced and is mostly insufficiently described in the literature on the subject. The art of conscious liberation from the poison of fear or the 'nobody loves me'-poison is the culmination of Hatha-Yoga.

THE ART OF THE DIRECTION OF WARMTH – SECOND ACT

In the previous sections the first phase of relaxation – the act of the sensation of heaviness – has been described. This is followed by the second act which is the sensation of warmth. But unlike in a play there is no interval between the two acts. Deep relaxation is a continuous process. Some scenes of the second act may already have taken place in the first act.

Students of relaxation will have experienced that a certain sensation of warmth occurs in the hands, the solar plexus or the space behind the eyes and, less often, in the feet. This usually happens when the first act changes over into the second act. A few students may find that any sensation of warmth begins in the solar plexus and not, as is the experience of most other people, in the extremities, spreading inwards from there. In this case the following route has to be redesigned. They must start with the solar plexus and direct the warmth from there to the extremities. Students who so far have not succeeded in experiencing any warmth at all (they usually are middle-aged or old people who are breathing badly) should always start with breathing exercises followed by their own physical 20-minute programme, and only then begin their relaxation. This means that they will have to devote about half an hour to Yoga. I think all students will profit from the following schedule because it simplifies the mental work during relaxation.

FIXING THE ROUTE

The decisive aspect of a timetable of any railway is regularity. The timetable tells us exactly at what time a train will depart and when it will arrive at its destination. This is only possible because the route has been fixed and the train does not encounter traffic jams which would call for redirection. The same applies with the mental processes during relaxation. There is only one way to facilitate relaxation, and this is by fixing the route along which the mind can travel securely and efficiently.

The route of relaxation begins with the toes and from there continues to the soles, insteps, ankles, calves, knees and thighs and the back. As we proceed along this route, the parts of the body along which we travel mentally become heavy. We then start with the fingers, palms, back of the hands, forearms, elbows, upper arms and shoulders. From there our mind moves down along the front and from the solar plexus into the abdomen. From there we return to the head, the point behind the eyes and finally the inside of the nose. In all these places we begin to experience the sensation of heaviness and first stirrings of warmth. The route also includes stops during which our mind concentrates on the breath. Then we arrive at the second act where we begin to feel how the body dissolves.

THE PILLAR EXPERIENCE

Relaxation is full of surprises. There is always the unexpected element which is of interest to a student exploring the mind. It seems that the experiences in deep relaxation are not the result of superimposed sensations but apparently are only triggered off by mental suggestions and grow from within. Thus for most beginners the experience of an overall fusion is completely new and surprising. This fusion consists in a melting together of hands, thighs or abdomen (according to where the hands are placed), or between heels, calves and knees to a single vibrating field, leading the student to the so-called pillar experience. His body becomes a structure without branches weighing tons and sinking deep into the ground. Buddhist Chinese literature describes this state of relaxation as a step towards meditation. They call it 'becoming like a tree'.

According to the Indian concept this stage of relaxation is a preparation for the withdrawal of the senses (*pratyahara*). For the advanced student this experience of fusion will lead to a strong sensation of warmth and then to a feeling of wholeness. He should make full use of this pillar experience in order to induce the sensation of warmth. The fusion of hands and feet belong to the programme of relaxation. It is possible to achieve the desirable warmth actively by way of invitation in order to direct it finally to any part of the body.

THE LAYING-ON OF HANDS

It is the most natural thing on earth that an ill person should place his hands on his abdomen if he suffers from colic or an attack of any other pain in that area. The hands radiate a certain warmth which is beneficial and soothing. One can experiment with this during the Contemplative Breath. If one breathes wrongly there will be hardly any warmth in the hands, but as soon as one starts with the rhythmic breathing one can experience a flow of heat from the hands into the body. This sensation is experienced by most students who have never heard or read about it before. The Indians say that deep breathing awakens something within us which is normally dormant. The laying-on of hands is a useful aid to the direction of warmth.

A higher form of this is the conscious direction of warmth through purely mental processes. This is the relaxation of a master which presupposes an active control over parts of the autonomic nervous system. Mental states induce physical processes like increased circulation and hence heightened activity of certain organs or glands over which we have otherwise no control. A master of Hatha-Yoga achieves this without any aids, but the beginner is permitted to assist his relaxation through friction with the use of a brush. Soon he will become independent of such means.

EXERCISE

Lie down on the floor and place cushions under head and arms as in the drawing. Cover yourself with a blanket. The hands frame the solar plexus. Close your eyes and begin with the Contemplative Breath in four bars. The inner organs sink back. Introspection. Darkness around the eyes. Then the sensation of warmth. Fusion of the limbs into a pillar-like structure. Increased warmth in the abdomen. Deep breathing. Slowly come back.

BLESSING OF THE WARMTH . . . NOT ONLY FOR COLD FEET

Besides framing the solar plexus with the hands, there are a number of other helps. One can, for example, place the hands

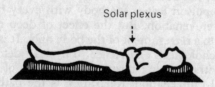

Solar plexus

Increased comfort with cushions supporting the arms

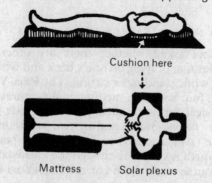

Cushion here

Mattress   Solar plexus

on a rebellious liver or a painful colon. The flow of heat to an arthritic hip which one touches with the hands can also be soothing. It is also possible and very desirable to direct this warmth down into our cold feet. The sensation of warmth in deep relaxation is the best and least expensive way of curing circulatory disturbances. No gadgets or drugs are required, merely the mental process of invitation and of opening up to the warmth. Physiologically speaking, this experience is a dilation of the blood vessels in the muscles and connective tissues, the organs and glands in skin and nerves. It is an indescribably pleasant sensation. The experience of warmth is the detoxication of the body as a conscious process.

WELL-BEING THROUGH REJUVENATION

We all experienced the flow of warmth when we were babies, and relaxation is a going back to this state of innocence and purity. The experience of warmth in relaxation acts as a bath which cleanses our bodies from all waste matter. One can really feel how the poison leaves the body with every breath. It is the path to rejuvenation. But the effect of deep relaxation is not confined to a refreshment of the body only. It is simultaneously a psychological experience. Physical detoxication is impossible without going through the process of mental and psychological rejuvenation. Relaxation is the path to a more introspective attitude of the mind and leads to an inner enrichment.

RELAXATION IN MEDITATIONAL POSTURES

I am sometimes asked whether there are other relaxation postures besides that of lying on one's back and whether a true Yogi can relax while standing or sitting. The Raja-Yogis distinguish between four so-called meditational postures. These are the three classical forms of sitting cross-legged; namely the Lotus posture (*padma-asana*) and its two variations, the Perfected posture (*siddha-asana*) and the Heroic posture (*vira-asana*). The fourth is strangely enough the Headstand (*shirsha-asana*). The course of discipline of the Raja-Yogi demands of him that he should be able to remain in any of these four postures for about three hours.

It is clear that few Western students will ever be able to do this. They will have to be satisfied with relaxing on their back. Even in India the beginner is recommended to assume this position. One reads sometimes that the Headstand is practised in order to relax. It would be more correct to call it a kind of refreshment, for deep relaxation is impossible in any position which requires continual balance, as one can never be completely passive and relax all the muscles. Of course partial relaxation can also be of great benefit. One question remains to be answered: Can relaxation be dangerous? All I can say is that deep relaxation is probably the only human activity from which no one has ever died.

Important: Relaxation teaches us to treat ourselves kindly. The student will find out that this does not come quickly. Setbacks are likely to occur. The most difficult pupils are those who do not even recognise that they are maltreating themselves. It is a common mistake among Western students not to protect their bodies after relaxation. It can be dangerous to take a cold shower or bath or expose oneself to draught.

THE STATE OF WHOLENESS

The reader will remember the diagram showing the relation between Hatha-Yoga and Raja-Yoga (see page 14). I now wish to say a few words about the 'window' in the wall which separates the two. An arrow points through the window. It indicates the important change which takes place when the student enters this borderline territory. For the third stage of relaxation leads into Raja-Yoga. This state is characterised by the experience of fusion. Soon we get the impression that the physiological phenomena recede more and more and give place to a kind of perfect reconciliation between body and mind. This leads to the experience of being no longer in the body. Finally there is the sensation of being elevated in a wonderful weightlessness. The student is much impressed by the sensation of floating, but this is only a side effect of the general feeling of wholeness.

TICKET TO THE MOUNTAIN PEAK

If we return again to the illustration of a schedule for deep relaxation, we will now imagine that our timetable is valid for a mountain railway with three stops. These correspond with the three stages of relaxation. Let us take the mountain train to the Piz Nair near St Moritz as an example. From St Moritz to Chantarella, with a difference of 200 metres in height, the ticket costs 1 franc. (Presumably more by now.) This stop corresponds with the experience of heaviness in relaxation. From Chantarella to Corviglia, which is 450 metres higher, one has to pay 3 francs. This stop corresponds with the experience of warmth during relaxation. Most passengers get out here and only a few are prepared to pay yet another 4 francs to go up to Piz Nair, which lies another 400 metres higher. The travellers who now and then reach the third stop are those who have paid the full price of the ticket by doing their exercises regularly every day. To get that far requires an inner readiness and acceptance of a certain measure of discipline. Not because someone else prescribes it, but from the sheer joy of exploring new territory. Perhaps you, too, will experience a quite unforeseen inner transformation.

COMPLETE HARMONY

It is not necessary, perhaps not even desirable, to put into words the experience on the deepest level of relaxation. I merely wish to indicate what reward a patient student can expect. In the third stage of relaxation body and mind are in complete harmony, accompanied by a perfect state of contentment. One experiences phenomena of light and might even hear unforgettable music.

Nature endows man with many talents. One may have perfect pitch, another a gift for painting and a third may be able to handle wild animals. The gift of relaxation, however, is common to all of us. That some people are able to relax less than others is not due to a lack of talent but to the resistance which they have built up. We should therefore have faith in this gift and regard the resistance as something temporary. It is important not to try to force the third stage.

Some readers who follow the advice contained in this book will have their first experience of wholeness when they suddenly awake from sleep and find that they breathe deep and rhythmically and enter an indescribably pleasant state of peace and fulfilment. This is a real blessing. It will not come to them unearned but still they may consider it as something which is given to them as a means to achieve harmony in themselves. From the many letters and personal accounts of my students it appears that all of them somehow felt that this experience was nothing really new but that they had been acquainted with it for a long time already.

REJUVENATION IN THIRTY DAYS

It is quite possible for Western students to experience an essential rejuvenation in a relatively short time. The change may be so drastic and convincing that it makes a great impression on everybody. How does one go about it? The secret of rejuvenation lies in having a clear programme and a definite goal. Success is the result of the daily practice. However, before one proceeds with making a programme for the rejuvenation in 30 days, one must be quite clear to what extent one can actually rely on one's own strength and how much one must count on the help of others such as one's doctor.

The following programme is meant as a suggestion for healthy people; they might be exhausted and in need of rest; they can be at the beginning of overweight but as long as they are not under medical treatment and heart, blood pressure and glands function normally, they are not really ill, merely in need of rejuvenation. Still, every student should seek medical advice before attempting to carry out this particular programme. To those who are ill or recovering from sickness I would like to say that Hatha-Yoga does not wish to replace the doctor, and a book about self-help through control of the body is far removed from being a textbook for self-diagnosis. These particular people should carry out their rejuvenation programme under medical supervision. The programme can be usefully combined with long walks, mountain tours or other forms of exercise. The healthy student best starts his rejuvenation programme during holidays.

Today rejuvenation is a widely recognised need which has given birth to big industries, extended advertising campaigns and a huge market of products. I do not wish to denigrate the value of certain articles, gadgets or methods. They apparently answer a demand. The teaching of Hatha-Yoga, however, is a response to the deep longing for genuine health. It is not a branded article. Its benefits are tremendous but have to be acquired through personal effort. It may be that the 30-day programme has to be repeated after a few years, but its effects are far-reaching and lasting.

PLANNING AND RESOLUTION

If someone only has the means for building a five-room house, he should not design a country mansion. The same applies to the 20-minute Yogi, who should realise his limitations. The resolution of the student is like a seed from which a huge tree may grow. If a gardener could harvest four weeks after sowing the seeds, he would make a very good business. The student who sticks to his programme for a month will make a similarly lucrative investment. Those who have experienced the results only once will keep to Yoga throughout their lives. The benefits derived from the 30-day programme will act as an incentive to go deeper into Yoga. What kind of results can be expected? The answer is—a beneficial detoxication of the body accompanied by deep peace, balance and the feeling of being young once more.

THE PROGRAMME—RESOLUTION

It is made in the understanding that for the next 30 days we will have to practise certain drastic disciplines in order to recuperate quickly. The 20-minute programme of Yoga is therefore done twice every day. Once in the morning before breakfast, once in the evening before dinner. The weight must be checked every day. For 30 days you should have a really filling breakfast and lunch but observe the rules for dinner according to the programme. For 30 days you should relax every day for at least 20 minutes. If it is impossible during the day, it has to be practised in the evening. However, it is part of the discipline not to exaggerate whatever you are doing.

PROGRAMME – DIET

The success or failure of the 30-day programme depends largely on the increase of excretion. It is not so important what you eat, but how quickly you get rid of it. In view of the fact that most people have to hold a job, a fasting cure is out of the question, but the rejuvenation is achieved through the combined effect of regular exercising and the avoidance of overburdening the stomach at night. That means that you have only fruit, a salad, and afterwards milk products for dinner. No bread, no potatoes or noodles, no sausages, butter or even margarine. No meat or fish. The fruit may be raw or cooked, fresh or dried according to season. It is possible to eat apples every night for the whole month. Dried fruit is better if it has been soaked first, but it should not be eaten by the pound. The daily ration of meat should be taken for breakfast or lunch. Breakfast must be the main meal. After three fruit meals in the evenings, hunger will undoubtedly come. There is no reason to avoid eggs or rice during the first two meals. No white bread, no smoking before breakfast.

These are 30 days of self-examination. How does my body react? How does it evacuate? How long does it take before a meal is digested? The goal is evacuation within 12 hours. Observe yourself how you stand, walk, lie, sit. Also observe your mental reactions and the changes in your emotional life as well as your vitality. Daily weighing. Those who are afraid of the scales will never slim. If after 30 days you succeed in wearing clothes of ten or more years ago, you have been rejuvenated by your own strength.

Then you can decide whether you wish to continue with your daily session of 20-minute Yoga.

Index

Note: figures in italics indicate that the pages referred to include diagrams